1

Look up to the sky. You'll never find the rainbows if you're looking down. 🌈

Charlie Chaplin

Look for the 'effin' rainbows. 🌈

Irene Wignall

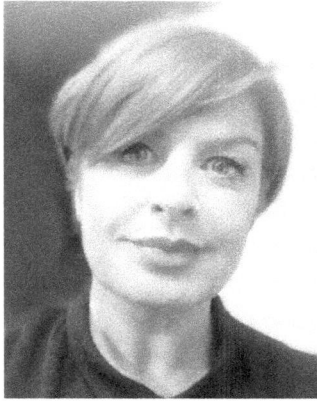

Irene Wignall is a new author who only attempted writing when she realised her head was full of randomness and she needed to off load some of it. When Irene started writing she was dealing with some very big events in her life and writing became like having a counselling session without the cost. Irene is a Detective in the Police, an amazing mum, an amazing wife and obviously writing this herself. She is 44 years old and lives in Bolton with her family. Irene's interests include wasting time on social media, repeating week three of couch to 5K every month and procrastinating.

For my stinks
Ted, Dusty and Albie
xxx

Contents

Preface

This book is about nothing and everything. This is definitely not a 'woe is me' kind of book and I'm not looking for sympathy. I love my life, the good and the bad -and the really ugly-. The things that I'm going to talk about are the things that have made me ... me.

I was raised in an ordinary family, as ordinary as most families are anyway. I was - and am - very loved by my parents and my two sisters. I am the eldest of the three of us. There's me, then four years later came my 'middle' little sister Catherine, then twenty years later, my 'little' little sister Hannah, who is taller than us all. We couldn't be more different, but as a unit, we're always there for each other, whether we're crying or laughing.

We weren't rich but we weren't on the breadline. School was non-eventful from what I remember. I wasn't bullied. I had a couple of fags on the playing fields, got a couple of detentions. I had best friends, I was happy.

When I was twelve years old I went into Bolton town centre with my friends and I was dared to steal a £4 bottle of white musk perfume from The Body Shop. I did it. Now, I believe in Karma but come on, it was only a £4 bottle of white musk. I apologise Mr Body Shop but I think I have paid my dues - and more - with the events I am going to tell you about.

My vision when I was growing up, was one of me, a husband and two little girls, wasn't too much to ask for, however, life had other ideas.

Growing Older is Inevitable, Growing Up is Optional

At twenty-five I still lived with my mum and my little-little sister, Hannah. When my friends came round to get ready before going out on the town, Hannah used to join us in the prinks, only hers was a Fruit Shoot. She'd put make up on like us and to be honest, she was probably better than us at it, even at that young age. When we set off, she was devastated we weren't taking her with us.

Catherine, my middle-little sister, had already moved out, and had a baby boy, Harry. She was already at the winging-it-at-motherhood stage. This, I later came to understand, is what we all are doing.

At around this same age, my mum had suggested that maybe I should look for somewhere to live; get on the property ladder. I was very comfortable at home, handing over a pittance as keep, out every weekend, new clothes, new cars, holidays. I loved to spend money, I still do, the only difference now is that I don't have any. I was very comfortable, who wouldn't be? However, grudgingly, I went to view one house, five minutes away - didn't want to venture too far into the big wide world - and bought it within weeks.

I made numerous trips to Ikea, which I loved and bought essentials: a spatula, love heart ice cube trays and lots of tea lights. The house was fully kitted out and I still hadn't moved in. Eventually, with some gentle coaxing, I made the big move and was happy there.

When I was twenty- six I married my on/off childhood sweetheart. We had been together for eleven years, but divorced after nine months when I was twenty-seven. We hadn't even got the wedding photos - this was before the digital age. My ex husband was my best friend for many years and it just seemed like a natural progression to get married, the thing to do. It's like when you start dating, you always get asked, 'when are you two going to get engaged?' then you do, and then it's, 'when's the wedding?' You get married, 'when's the babies?' You have one and then you're asked, 'when are you having another one?' and so on. Woah there, let's just enjoy one moment at a time - enjoying the moment I'm in is something I struggle with.

We had the big Irish wedding, but in Bolton. A two day affair, a great weekend, but I knew I was kidding myself. There were hundreds of people there, half of them I didn't even know. It was around this time that I started to discover there were more people out there and perhaps my best friend of eleven years wasn't my soul mate after all. The timing could have been a tad better. Suffice to say, it was all my fault, and between the ages of twenty-seven and thirty- two, I was living my life in the way I should have done before I walked down any aisle.

I met my now husband Adam at the age of thirty-two. Strangely, I think this is the age I became an adult and my morals re-appeared. The years between twenty-seven and thirty-two could be a Bridget Jones novel all on their own. Some of which I could print, most of it I couldn't, unless I wrote under a pseudonym. A lot I can't remember or chose to block out - or black out...

Speaking of black outs, I was - as were most of my friends - a binge drinker. I went out to get drunk and meet the man of my dreams. Surely, I was going to find the man of my dreams after five Sambucas, a few cheeky Vimtos, followed by a kebab? What a catch I was, struggling to stand, unable to speak any sense and thinking I looked amazing, dancing to I'm a Dreamer in the local club.

On my 30th birthday night out I lost one single gold shoe. Think Cinderella, only, I found my shoe the next day myself, wearing my Uggs and last night's make up, no handsome prince featured. On many nights I lost my purse and keys and had to break into my house. I was a dab hand at it in the end. Maybe a new career choice?

I once rang my mum from Manchester crying. I was drunk and couldn't get home. Unfortunately, drunk-me must have forgotten I was upset because I decided to go back to a club and forgot she was on her way for me - sorry mum.

I phoned up the bank one Sunday morning, devastated as my bank card had been stolen. I spoke to 'Alan' on the help-line, a man with a strong Indian accent.

'Hi,' I said, 'I've had my bank card stolen.'
'Okay where did you last use it?'
'Last night, about eight o'clock, on my way into town.'
'Okay, could it have been outside Wetherspoons around 3am where you put your pin number in wrong three times, so your card was taken?'
Hmmm?
'Thanks for your help, Alan.'

At the end of these drunken nights, I somehow always got the same taxi driver and in my drunken haze we discovered he used to work with my mum. This taxi driver saw me at my worst. I probably over-paid him on numerous occasions when I still had my purse with me at the end of the night and I doubtless under-paid him too. He may even have broken into my house with me. I told him my biggest secrets, he was like my hairdresser but when I was drunk. I was in the gym one evening pretending I was a health freak, not a massive lush who couldn't usually remember the end of the night, when I turned to see Mr Taxi Driver waving at me through the glass doors. OMG, I didn't want to mix my drunk-life with my pretend-healthy-life. It felt like seeing someone I had drunkenly slept with waving at me in the gym. I couldn't get out of there quick enough. Poor bloke, he was just being friendly.

My dating life was a laughable series of unfortunate events at this time. Here are a few highlights/lowlights just to give you an idea:

- I once went for a curry with a bloke I met in a club and he said something to offend me - obviously it must have been really bad as I can't remember what that something was - so I threw a glass of water over him. Feeling very Carrie Bradshaw-esque and pleased with myself, I stood up to walk out just as he threw the full jug of water over me ... that's not how it happens to Carrie. I wish I'd gone for the jug first.

- I went out with a man who had just done ten years for armed robbery. I should have realised something wasn't right when he was clearly wearing someone else's trousers. In fact, he was wearing tuxedo trousers with a satin stripe down the side of each leg, which were about six inches too short. But, he was fit, so I told myself I'm all about rehabilitation and forgiving people who've paid their dues. I should mention that I am a detective in the police and have been for twenty years, so maybe not my ideal soul mate option.

- I went on a blind date with someone who I was told looked like Orlando Bloom. Unfortunately, he looked more like Jesus with bulging thumbs.

- I dated a man who lived with his wife but they were separated and they didn't love each other anymore. Really, Irene?

- I dated a man who was a health freak during a time where I was on first name terms with the local pizza man. The pizza man who told me one day when he was delivering my pizza that I was only allowed one a week.. The health freak also once went through my bins whilst I was out to see if I had ordered pizza that week, I don't need that kind of pressure... Next.

Introducing myself to strangers in these clubbing days caused me anxiety. In my younger years at school I loved the fact that I was the only Irene, but when it came to meeting blokes on a night out it was a different story. I would have various retorts after telling them my name: 'Are you serious?' 'Wow, that's a granny's name'. It didn't help when the only Rita in my year at school changed her name to Jañe. Should I change my name? What would I change it to? Something exotic? As I clearly looked exotic with my pale skin, blue-green eyes and a strong northern accent.

Now I'm older, I'm glad I never changed my name. I am unique - apart from in an old people's home where we are ten to a penny. Plus when, Come on, Eileen comes on, I think I'm cool and dance in the middle of my friends pretending the song is about me.

Three things that I am grateful for;

- **Finding my gold shoe**
- **Dating a fit bloke, regardless of his rap sheet**
- **I'm still best mates with the pizza man**

Finding my Mr Big… who turned out to be my Mr Tall

Adam and I worked at the same police stations, he was in uniform and I was in C.I.D. we knew of each other but had never really had a conversation. I was night detective one shift, which meant you were the only detective on that night and Adam came up to me for some advice with a job he was dealing with. Adam is 6" 5' which I love, and he is confident without the arrogance, most of the time. I remember thinking as we chatted over the job, he's actually really nice, so I was brave and gave him my personal telephone number if he ever needed any more advice. In my head this meant, 'here's my number ask me out'. A couple of days later Adam rang me. I knew it! However, he was just letting me know the outcome of the job. Yes, cheers Adam...

I know now that if I want Adam to do something I need to say exactly what I want, not to wait to see if he can read my mind, because he can't.

Our paths didn't cross again until eighteen months later when I bumped into him in Crown Court. I noticed him straightaway amongst the group of cops, probably as he was about a foot taller than anyone else. We spoke briefly then a couple of days later I thought, I'm going to ask him out. This is something I had never done, well at least not when sober. Obviously I wasn't going to ask him out like a grown-up, face to face, I needed a safety net so I texted him and had to wait a full thirty mins for his reply. *Are you kidding me?*

This is bit of a cliché but on our first date I knew I would marry him and have children with him. I even told the taxi driver on my way home. I thought I'd let Adam know a few dates down the line - don't want to be showing all your crazy straightaway, ladies. On our date, I wore jeans and boots. Unbeknownst to Adam, I had cut off the bottom of my jeans so they would fit in my boots. My ulterior motive was so that I would be sensible and go home on my own on our first date. Not my proudest hour having to ruin a good pair of jeans so I didn't sleep with him. But, as I said, I was now entering my adulthood and that seemed a very grown up thing to do. And I wanted to marry Adam.

On our date every time I went to the toilet or bar Adam would turn and watch me walk back. Wow, I thought, he must really fancy me, he can't keep his eyes off me. It was only later he told me he was going bald at the back and didn't want me to notice. The things we do …

The week after our date we were both very much into each other. Adam told me he had a son called Callum who was three years old. In my head I thought, fertile - tick. But I didn't vocalise that thought. We texted each other constantly throughout the week. Then much to my surprise he said he would ring me on his break. What? An actual phone conversation? I can do texts; I'm funny in texts but an actual conversation? I went into panic mode. I got some post-it-notes - I love post-it-notes - and wrote down topics of conversation we could talk about. This was me - an adult, thirty-two years of age with one marriage already behind me. I ticked off each topic as we went along and we had a lovely conversation if not exactly free flowing. I told him about the post-its two years later.

I guess my gut was right with this one, because years later, Adam is one of the most laid back people I know, and I am … how should I put it? Not. He likens us to Pamela and Mick from Gavin and Stacy just without the Charles and Camilla role playing.

What Adam failed to tell me about, but I what I quickly experienced, were his night terrors. (Clearly not until after the third date, I do have rules now.) The first night it occurred I was fast asleep at his flat when he jumped up out of bed screaming like a girl. He looked like he was knocking things off him. Later it came to light, he was hitting at spiders. This was a regular occurrence. I decided to download an app that started recording as soon as it detected any noise. I was woken one night with Adam sat astride me with a pillow in his hands, ready to put it over my face, I slapped him hard across the face and he shouted, 'What was that for?'

"Erm Adam, that was because you were trying to kill me.'

Each morning we'd eagerly press play to see what it had recorded. One morning, we heard Adam say, 'Is this Irene?' Another morning he said, 'Piss on me'. Our big grins froze and our excitement waivered as we suddenly didn't find the recordings that amusing. I stopped recording after this as it wasn't funny-cute anymore just funny-weird, also it seemed like I may be creating a defence for him if he 'accidently' killed me.

Things I am grateful for;

- **Being brave enough to ask Adam**
- **Post it notes**
- **Cutting the bottom off my jeans**

Move over Mary Berry

We are chalk and cheese, but it works. I try to be the perfect wife, but it often gets lost in translation. To say I'm not particularly into cooking would be an understatement. One day, I was off work and Adam was on a twelve-hour shift. The dutiful wife would have his dinner on the table as he walked in, so I thought I'd give it a go. I'd love to be one of those people who opens the cupboard and sees X, Y and Z and thinks that will make A. However, I'm not. I looked in the cupboard and saw a jar of Korma curry sauce and pasta. I looked in the fridge for more inspiration and saw pickled onions. Voila! Korma pasta! Made with the pickled onions as I had no real onions. He came in and saw the feast and said in shock, 'what is that?' Personally, I don't know how he could not see it was Korma Pasta. Suffice to say it went in the bin and Adam cooks now.

Now that Adam does the cooking, the kitchen looks like a bombsight every evening. He likes to prep everything first then put all the ingredients into separate bowls like he's some sort of Jamie Oliver. He even does this even with cheese on toast. I can't have everything I suppose. I bought a dish washer.

On this note, even though I'm not the greatest cook, he is terrible at D.I.Y. He was putting up a light fitting in our lounge when I advised him the light should be flush with the ceiling and his reply was, 'Look at you making words up'. So I have a man I pay by the hour. We can't all be great at everything.

He does have his good points. Adam always comments if I've had my hair cut or nails done. I recently went to have a pamper, to spend some quality time on my own, rather than walking round Tesco's aimlessly. When I arrived home calm, serene and beautified, Adam commented on how lovely I looked.

'Thanks Adam, what have I had done?'

'You've had your eyelashes trimmed.'

No women in the world, Adam, would ever get her eyelashes trimmed but ten out of ten for effort.

Things I am grateful for;

- **Not having to cook anymore**
- **Finding a man who's handy, even if I have to pay him**
- **Never having to have my eye lashes trimmed**

What to expect when you're … not expecting

I had always wanted babies but had no age in mind and, before Adam came along, no bloke in mind either. My middle sister, Catherine, had Harry, my nephew, when she was eighteen, so I always borrowed him when I felt broody. It was a great situation as Catherine was still young and wanted to see her friends and I was happy to get my baby-fix. It sort of came to a head when I lost Harry. I don't think she trusted me so much after that. Harry was at mine for the day and I was suffering from a hangover but also wanted my Harry-fix. He must have been around three years old at the time. We were in my bedroom while I hung up the clothes strewn around from the previous night and I felt quite sleepy. 'I know what Harry, let's have a nap.' I know now just because I want a nap you can't make a three-year-old nap …

I woke up twenty minutes later and Harry was gone. I called his name. Nothing. I ran downstairs, the door was closed, so he couldn't have got out, could he? I searched outside shouting him. Shit, I had literally lost my nephew. It seemed like an age but in reality it was about twenty minutes later that I thought, Right, this shit is getting serious, I best call my mum. I got my mum out of a meeting and she got straight in the car to come to mine.

I rang Catherine. 'Catherine, I'm really sorry but I've lost Harry.' Catherine immediately got a taxi and spent the journey hysterically crying to the taxi driver who advised her not to let me look after Harry again. Which I suppose is fair enough. Everyone was on their way and I sat on my bedroom floor crying. Nothing for it but to call the police. I reached for my phone and glanced under my bed and there was Harry fast asleep. Oh, how we laughed … ten years later when we had all gotten over the shock of it all and I had been forgiven.

Catherine got pregnant again about seven years after having Harry and I cried when she told me. I was happy for her, but it should have been me next. There I was dating with no sign of a 'baby-daddy' in sight. She miscarried, and I have always blamed myself that my selfish thoughts caused it.

Catherine and I are on opposite sides of the spectrum. Catherine is dizzy and doesn't plan anything. She would be bored to tears if she had my life. And my head would pop off if I had hers. We both respect that we are different and we have great times together. Most of our laughs are at her mishaps. They make me feel intelligent.

- She was on a course from work one day and one of the first questions on the welcome form was gender and she asked her colleague what they were putting.

- On my fortieth birthday party she set fire to her hair, possibly I was partly to blame with my love of tea lights.

- She joined in a serious discussion recently about boycotting chocolate spread due to the orangutans. Catherine said, 'No way is chocolate spread made from orangutans?'

No words …
But I suppose me losing her son sort of tops all those.

Things with Adam moved fast we started trying for a family. I was convinced given my age of thirty-four that we would have problems, so much so that we did have problems. I believe I created these issues myself. All the self-help books about positivity that I've read since then state that you receive what you put out into the universe, and what I was emitting was, 'time is running out'. I think my insides sensed my panic and decided they'd become hostile.

I wanted to give up smoking before I got pregnant, so I attended a cessation class. The two things that struck me were, how miserable everyone was, and how god-damn wrinkly the women looked. Never mind my lungs, I did not want wrinkles like that, so I stopped smoking. I would be pregnant soon anyway, so I couldn't smoke then. They should put photos of women's mouths looking like a cat's arse on the front of cigarette packets as opposed to some black lungs and I'm sure the government would see a significant decline in smoking.

After eighteen months of trying and a timetable of 'when to have sex' and no cigarettes, we were still baby-less.

We were referred to the fertility clinic. I couldn't help but find it hilarious that Adam had to provide a sample - I'm very mature. However, Adam already had Callum so I was sure the issue wasn't with him.

After a few months and multiple tests later, I was prescribed Chlomid. This is a tablet that helps your body release more eggs and can potentially result in multiple births. We had three months' worth to start.

After the first month, I had to go for a scan to ensure the Chlomid was doing what it needed to do. The doctors found some issue that meant I had to stay overnight at the hospital. I can't even remember what the problem was now but at the time I couldn't stop crying. I had never stayed in hospital overnight and even at thirty-five, it was scary. In an act of divine irony, that same day one of my many cousins in Ireland, had a baby. It wasn't that much of a sign; with thirty-four first cousins it was likely that one of us would be having a baby at any given moment.

The next morning a lovely doctor came in and said 'We have some good news. You're pregnant.'

I was ecstatic and I couldn't wait to get out of the hospital. They told me I had to go back in a couple of days later for more blood tests, but I was more than okay with that. I was so excited I didn't even wait for Adam to collect me. I started walking home, literally skipping out of the hospital. I'd already worked out when the baby would be due, her birth sign, Aquarius, and to be honest with you, I'd probably decided her coming-home outfit from the hospital. Can one day old babies wear shoes? Surely they can. Where's my credit card?

After telling no one apart from everyone, I had a call from the hospital on the Thursday. They explained to me that the pregnancy hormone levels were going down, so I was not pregnant and I must have had an early miscarriage the month before. Great, cheers for that.

That must be my Karma paid back now?

I had to go back to the hospital the following Monday for more blood tests. A doctor came in, a skinny-looking Asian man with zero bed-side manner. He didn't even make eye contact. It was clear I was just another buff-coloured file to him. I could have forgiven all that, but after he walked in, he exclaimed, 'Congratulations you're pregnant.'

Through gritted teeth I asked, 'Is this the same pregnancy I had last week that wasn't a pregnancy or is this a new one?'

Then he shuffled through his notes and said, 'Oh yes, you're not pregnant.' What a tosser.

I've met a lot of Consultants and Doctors in my adult life, and as much as I admire them for what they do, empathy is not something that I've found is high on their list of qualifications. But I suppose it may be a mechanism for self-preservation?

-P.S. I am very grateful to the NHS in the following years-

Things I am grateful for;

Actually getting pregnant

The NHS in a sort of way

Being brave in hospital

New House, New Mindset

During the same month, Adam and I picked a house and moved in together. I say 'we' picked a house, I mean I. I'm a big fan of Right Move. I filtered through hundreds of houses, discounted them, and showed Adam just two houses. He thinks it was easy, picking our house, little did he know the hours upon hours of research I'd done, and if truth be told, continue to do just in case we win the lottery.

It was so exciting. I had a flip chart and signs on each box. I was in my element. My family call me Monica, from Friends. If there is a way to incorporate a filing system, a planning system, spreadsheets or highlighters into an activity, you can bet I will do it. Just buying a new planner for the year takes a lot of research.

On the same weekend we moved into our new house, Adam had committed to walking a Night Marathon in memory of his friend's fiancée who had sadly passed away. In the recesses of my mind I remembered that someone had told me something about marathon runners and Vaseline, so, me being a caring partner, relayed this and told Adam to put some Vaseline on his feet. Unfortunately, I remembered the advice incorrectly, and the Vaseline should have been on his nipples so they didn't chafe. Rubbing his feet in slippery Vaseline made them slide about in his shoes and within about 3 miles he was suffering with blisters and struggling to walk. Oops.

When he came back to our new home he couldn't walk. Our new house was a town house, so he had two flights of stairs to climb to get to our bedroom. He eventually got to the bedroom and asked me to help him. I filled a bowl full of water, put it at the side of the bed and went out. I would never make a very good nurse. In my head, I was being caring because listening to him moaning and groaning made me want to punch him, but I didn't. I was thinking about him by going out. How kind am I?

He often says he would be worried if he was seriously ill as I would be nowhere in sight. I don't pretend that I will be. Might as well be honest from the start.

As our house was a new build, we had no fences in the back garden. I did some research and found a man. I was at work when he arrived with just a spade over his shoulder. That should have rung alarm bells. I was even more worried when Adam rang to tell me our fence man was asking Adam how he should do it. Adam rang me later in the day saying the fence man was now showing him Karate moves.

When I got home from work and walked into the garden, the fence looked the part. It was only when I looked out of the bedroom window bedroom that I saw he had built the fence around the rocks and rubble that were in his way. It was a snake shape rather than a straight line. It was only then that I read the fence guy's reviews properly. None of them mentioned his actual work, they just said, 'he's a lovely bloke'. You live and learn, and at least the fence is unique.

Actually, I don't live and learn. I was collecting a kebab one evening and there on the counter was a business card for a bathroom fitter. No research, I booked him. Another mistake; he broke everything he touched meaning it cost double to get the work done. I like to read the reviews now not just skim them, and I leave the business cards that I find on kebab shop counters well alone.

We now had a four-bedroom house to fill and a Ford Focus for our family car. I've always loved cars. To me, they represent each period of my life. My first car was a C Registered Fiesta in Maroon, it died when I drove through a puddle. I've had other cars and a couple of convertibles in my younger years, but I wanted a sensible family car when we tried for babies. I began to resent the Ford Focus as it represented what I didn't have. Now I have a VW Beetle with not much room for kids in the back, I'm not sure what that says about me.

Eventually three months of Chlomid had gone by, and still no baby, so the doctors decided to give us a month break, and then put us on a higher dosage before we went down the IVF route. Adam was petrified at the thought of me getting the higher dose as he really did not want twins or triplets. Me on the other hand. How hard could triplets be? I start ed googling multiple births. We could have our own TV program if there were seven of them and people would donate a van surely?

During our stress-free month off, with the help of normal unplanned sex, two comedy events - Steve Merchant on the Friday night and Dave Spikey on the Saturday night - lots of laughing - and sperm - I conceived. I knew I felt different. If you have ever tried for babies, Google is your best friend and worst enemy. Searches like, 'what's the earliest time a test can detect pregnancy?' and, 'what do you feel when you are pregnant?' and, 'can you start craving Mars Bars on day one of pregnancy?'

I bought a pregnancy test, and, in my urgency, I peed on the wrong end. Great start. Then Adam had to go to work so I agreed to get another test and we'd try again the next morning, a full 24 hours later, 1440 minutes, 86400 seconds. Not that I was counting.

I'm not a very patient person, and by not very I mean not at all. I would have loved to be able to tell you I waited for me and Adam to do it together, sitting on the floor in our bathroom that cost twice as much as it should have done, hugging and crying when we saw the second line, but sack that shit I needed to know. I got another test on my way to work, peed on the right end this time, and with my best friend in the office toilets, at nine am, we both waiting apprehensively for the second blue line. I was pregnant.

That evening ironically, Adam and I were meeting at a potential wedding venue, so that's when I first saw Adam having learnt I was pregnant. Everything was falling into place. We were shown around the venue and booked it for December 30th, 2012, (although he hadn't officially asked me to marry him) five months after our baby was due to arrive. This was my first time meeting the venue manager who showed us around and I blurted out that I was pregnant because I was just so eager to tell people. I felt a bit of a tit when she asked how far on I was.

We decided to make a weekend of it going looking for potential engagement rings. That also didn't go as planned. I had seen a lovely shop in Windermere in the Lake District that had rings that were just a little different. We booked a night in a hotel and planned the romantic trip. We walked into the town straight to the shop to look. I pointed at one straight away, 'that's it, that's the one'. However, Adam just looked at the price and went mad. We ended up having a row on the street and going back to the Hotel. We continued to not speak whilst at the hotel and X Factor came on. I explained to Adam I would talk to him about X Factor and X Factor only, then when the program finished I would go back to not speaking. I know, I'm very mature.

This should have been a warning sign to Adam, but he just put this down to a rare irrational blip. Ha! Little did he know.

A few weeks later I asked Adam if he had ordered the ring - we were talking again by this stage - I love surprises but I also ruin any surprise Adam tries to carry out due to being impatient. He told me the ring was coming from their shop in Brussels and there was a delay. Oh, right, that's okay then. Laptop out, googled the shop to find their Brussels' branch. No such thing, he had the ring all along, all I had to do now was act surprised. I had to make a conscious effort each day to stop myself from screaming to him, 'Just give me the god dam ring'.

I had my nails done in anticipation for my 'surprise'. Bonfire Night he suggested we get some fireworks and go to a lovely place near our new home. He knows I like Bonfire Night, so I knew it was going to happen. Act surprised Irene, act surprised. He asked me. I burst out crying.

He still thinks I was none the wiser. Until he reads this that is.

Three things I am grateful for;

🌈   **Getting pregnant again**
🌈   **Comedy events**
🌈   **Getting my nails done for my 'surprise' proposal**

The Pregnancy Glow

Five days into being pregnant and I'd told my boss - in confidence - and everyone I bumped into in those five days, in confidence. I started planning, as that is my forte. My little girl would be chubby - like me - but gorgeous, funny and have curly hair. I was dying to buy clothes but resisted. We would go shopping together, we would moan when daddy pumped or picked his nose. Me and my girl were going to be best friends.

We had agreed not to find out the sex. And I was okay with that, right up until the moment when the sonographer said, 'Do you want to know the sex?' Before Adam could answer, I blurted, 'Yes'.

'You're having a little boy.' She replied.

A boy? Check again. I can't do boys, they stink, fart, burp, they don't do cute things, they wear rubbish clothes. I hate to admit this, but I started crying and I couldn't stop. I had to lie to the sonographer and say they were happy tears, but I knew they weren't and so did Adam. My dream of a baby girl all in pink with curls smiling at me faded away. That is not what I had planned, envisaged, seen in my head. What the fuck do I do with a boy? In hindsight it was a good thing that I found out, so I could prepare myself for having a boy and not do all the crying when he arrived.

During my pregnancy I ate a lot, I also had raging hormones. I was in Asda getting my 'big shop' when I clocked the young lad serving me, he was gorgeous, but half my age, I was blushing. I phoned my little sister to explain to her I had found her future husband. At least then I could look from afar. Oh god, what had I become?

I read the last volume of Fifty Shades of Grey, this didn't help with my pregnancy hormones. We had decided as soon as we knew our baby was a boy he was going to be called Ted as we couldn't agree on any other boy's names, I had lots of girl names obviously. When I got to the last chapter of Fifty Shades I was devastated, they called their child Theodore. I was inconsolable; crying to Adam, spluttering that everyone was going to call their newborns Ted now. Pregnancy may have made me a tiny bit emotional.

Adam said I looked gorgeous throughout my pregnancy but wasn't into having sex in case he poked the baby's head. Now I'm not calling Adam's manhood, but I can assure you that wasn't going to happen. I asked Adam daily did I look fat to which he replied I looked gorgeous and no, I was not fat. Looking back at photos I couldn't even open my eyes properly my cheeks were that fat. But I'll forgive him as I didn't want to hear how fat I was getting. I could see it myself - just about with my slitty eyes.

That fact that the Fifty Shades books were released in 2011 meant there was a baby boom in 2012. How mental that a book can affect the population numbers. When Ted eventually started school, there was a double intake. I sometimes look at the mums in the playground thinking, did we all got horny and conceive whilst reading Fifty Shades of Grey?

I had a pregnancy book that I journaled throughout the nine months, that we have never looked at since. I read the Folk of the Faraway Tree to my growing belly, how dare they change the names of the main characters Fanny and Dick to Franny and Rick, I mean, Rick, what kind of enchanted forest name was that?

I had a bell on a long chain, so Ted could hear it, I listened to classical music in my car. I bored everyone to death what size he was: 'now he's the size of a pumpkin seed, now he's a walnut', like I was the only person ever to have gotten pregnant. I enjoyed being pregnant. People smiled at me for no reason other than I had growing belly. I felt like a walking miracle.

Three things I am grateful for;

- **Being told I was having a healthy baby**
- **The sonographer not realising how shallow I actually was**
- **Having a Bo... being told my baby was healthy.**

How to lose two and a half stone in ten days

Ted's delivery was far from plain sailing, and the process gave me Sepsis so I never saw him arrive and I didn't see him for a full thirty-six hours. Again, this is not how I planned it - are you sensing the theme in my life?. In my head, my waters would break, I would instantly start groaning, nip to hospital and he would arrive and be placed on my chest and immediately start breast feeding and my stomach would go back to an ironing board - that I never had in the first place. That's the least he could do since he already did me the disservice of not being a little girl. Although give him his due, with me having Sepsis I did lose two and a half stone in the first ten days, of the five stone I had put on, may I add.

But, my reality was that my waters broke early in the morning then nothing happened for the next day and a half. A midwife came to my house and did a sweep. I know you lose all your dignity when you're having a baby but having a sweep made me feel like a pregnant fat cow with a vet's arm up my vagina.

The sweep failed so I was booked in to be induced. She gave me a choice of which day I wanted. This wasn't something I could rush into - what's the rhyme about babies born on specific days of the week? I needed to make sure I didn't give birth on a Wednesday or my boy would have been full of woe. So, I picked a Thursday, he would have far to go. I took this to mean a long life ahead. Honestly, the way my mind works is a little bit scary.

I got to the hospital on Thursday morning ready to have my baby. I was sick and my waters broke fully all over the ward floor. I had a few midwives examining the content of my waters on the floor - a bit of a strange scenario - and they decided they were cloudy, everything seemed to be hurried along then.

They were monitoring Ted's heart rate and mine. My heart rate increased rapidly, and my legs started to shake, funny I hadn't heard of this happening in my antenatal classes. I then had to sign a form saying that I was the priority and they needed to save me first. My mum and Adam were rushed out and I was on my own. Was this in my birthing plan? This was all a blur and I didn't have any time to panic, I was anesthetised.

I woke up from the anaesthesia, and I'm not soft with pain but my God, I literally felt like I had been run over by a bus. I wasn't allowed any pain relief until I had fully come around, and by God could you tell when I had fully come around, screaming like a banshee.

Adam had shown me a photo of Ted. I was annoyed that he had gone to see him before me, our baby boy had a mass of brown hair and a little chin and little forehead like me. Adam asked if I minded if he went to sit with Ted as he had no one with him. Well, this was a new feeling; a little person who'd I not even met being a priority over me. I wasn't quite sure about how I felt about this but didn't want to come across like a petulant child in front of witnesses.

I was taken to a recovery ward where I had a nurse assigned to me. I was wearing an oxygen mask and my lips were so dry. I remembered I had brought my Elizabeth Arden Eight Hour Cream in my bag, along with my makeup and a book. Adam got the cream for me, when the nurse came back I was nicely glossed up, when she barked, 'what have you got on your lips?' She was fuming. I had to wipe it off. I felt like I had been caught wearing lipstick by my form teacher. How was I to know the oxygen would react with the cream and burn my lips?

After a few hours I was moved to a ward with three other women and their babies. Ted was in the Special Care Baby Unit. As I didn't have a baby beside me like the others, Adam bought me an enormous Teddy bear and he sat it by my side instead, he was Ted Two. I went to visit Ted One and I couldn't deny he was cute, so I was warming to him. It may have been because it was like looking in a mirror. I had never seen a baby look as much like his mother. We both had the same size foreheads. I'm not blessed in the forehead department, I have more of a two head and I'm okay with this.

I was so wrecked, the nurses kept ringing up the ward I was on, saying, 'your baby's crying can you come down and feed him?' Are you serious. I'm poorly here and very tired. But I know now that no matter how I'm feeling if my children need me it's tough shit and I have to go. I walked slowly down to the Special Baby Unit to delay trying to breast feed him.

After his birth I expected this wave of love to come over me and it just didn't come. I started to be hit with the panicked thought of, oh my god after all this I'm not a natural mum. With Ted spending a few days in the Special Care Unit it was like a mini boot-camp. When he was reunited with me he was good as gold and hardly made a sound. I tried breastfeeding but that was a joke. I tried believe me. There I was sat in the hospital bed with no top on, my boobs massive with veins running through them, my belly massive with stretch marks running through it, and the midwife saying, 'hold him like a rugby ball'.

My dad sat opposite me, watching me manhandling my

massive boobs trying to get Ted latched on, crying. My Dad reassuringly saying, 'you can do it, love, you can do it'.

The day I fell in love unconditionally with Ted was the day I gave him his first bottle. It was about 3am and I had had enough. I asked one of the other new mums for some bottled formula. She could see I was on the edge, she handed over a couple to keep Ted going until Adam arrived later that morning.

I gave Ted the bottle of formula, we both looked into each other's eyes with no stress, no boobs, no rugby balls and no crying. Just love. At that moment, Ted and I became firm best friends.

After ten very hot July days in the hospital, they finally let me out. I had Ted's going home outfit ready. I had bought it when I was maybe two hours pregnant. It was a pair of shorts, a shirt and cute shoes. What else could a new born baby want for comfort? I think they lasted ten minutes. The shoes were balanced on the end of his feet for just enough time for me to take a photo and get it on Facebook, obviously I needed to make sure I looked like a dab hand at this motherhood thing on social media. Now I'm writing a book to expose it all …

I was home for one day and night, but I was struggling to breath. I couldn't finish a sentence without pausing and taking a deep breath. I couldn't lie flat either. The first night I was home I was sat up in bed trying to get some sleep with Adam. Ted was in his Moses basket at the side of me. I said to Adam, "if I die in the night will you explain to the paramedics that I couldn't breathe properly?' Adam just ignored me and rolled over to sleep. The midwife came the next day, but after watching me struggling to breathe whilst talking to her she sent me back to the hospital.

Thankfully Ted could come back with me. Once in hospital I had scan after scan, I was booked in for a scan on my lungs Friday afternoon and the consultant had said if it comes back clear then I can go home before the weekend. A porter came to wheel me down to the scan, I could walk, but I took the ride anyway. Once in the scan room, the radiographer said, 'okay I'm going to be scanning your legs',

'Erm no, you're scanning my lungs.' I replied.

He went on to say, 'that's not what it says here, and I have to go off what it says'.

I started crying with sheer frustration. 'Just ring the effing consultant and ask!'

He refused and went onto scan my legs. I didn't wait for the porter on the way back, I stormed back into the maternity ward, shouting and crying at the midwife. That was my scanning slot gone - I was in for the weekend. Monday morning eventually arrived and after my lung scan it turned out that I just had forgotten how to breathe properly and needed physiotherapy to get back breathing again.

Wow, how do you forget how to breath?

Three things I am grateful for;

Remembering how to breathe again

Ted being healthy

My Dad being brave watching me manhandling my boobs

A Boy's Best Friend is his Mummy

After reading all the Annabelle Karmel books, The Baby whisperer and lots more on weaning babies, I'd vowed to only use fresh food made by my 'capable' hands. Ted only drank water. No sugar would pass his lips till he was at least ten.

I'd read somewhere to introduce spices and a variety of foods into his diet early on, so I purchased a steamer, as that's what Google said I needed and who was I to argue? I steamed loads of vegetables and decided to add some garlic. I grated it up on the freshly steamed goodness and proceeded to give to Ted. With each mouthful he gagged. I thought this was fine; he could get used to the taste of garlic and we'd move onto the next spice. At the same time, my dad rang, he very rarely rings me. Our talks usually go like this, 'hi, how you are doing? Is my mum there?' But this time I went on to tell my dad about what Ted was eating and him gagging at every mouthful. Dad's culinary delights consist of spam, mash and beans, and corned beef hash, so I though he may be impressed as Ted wasn't having Korma Pasta. But my Dad asked, 'Have you cooked the garlic?'

'Erm no? Should I have done?' No wonder Ted was gagging. Sorry Ted. I tried.

I enrolled in all the baby classes I could find: baby massage, baby yoga, baby rock and roll. My only problem was I wasn't very good at talking baby talk all the time, so I looked like a right miserable git sat having toast at snack time, me and Ted huddled in a corner not making eye contact with anyone. Maybe if I had made eye contact, I would have realised that we were all winging it, and nobody had a clue?

Soon, Ted had moved on to the rolling stage and fell off the bed on five occasions. It wasn't until my mum said, 'maybe you shouldn't leave him on the bed anymore?' that I stopped leaving him on the bed. I'd like to think of myself as fairly intelligent, but these basic thoughts seemed to bypass my brain at this time.

Each week I religiously went to get Ted weighed and then proceeded to text all my family to tell them what he weighed. It was like I was the only mother to ever have a baby grow. My family, bless them, feigned their interest. When Ted started hitting the ninety-percentile range on the growth chart I stopped taking him through fear I'd be judged. We didn't need that kind of negativity on our lives.

Ted had big hair right from the word go. He had a mass of curls which I loved. We decided we wouldn't cut his hair and let it just grown naturally. Each stage we went through we loved and thought he just looked the cutest. It wasn't until we looked back on photos that we realised it just looked like a nest. I suppose it's a parent's denial, like if you have an ugly child but you don't see it.

We booked Ted's christening for his first birthday. We aren't particularly religious but I was brought up Catholic and I wanted to cover all bases in case anything ever happened. Plus the only good secondary school near us was a Catholic school. I wanted everything to be perfect. My mother in law had given us Adam's christening shawl to use and everything was meticulously planned. I was running round the house like a crazed woman, trying to get Ted and myself ready and Adam and Callum were playing football outside. Adam says it only takes him ten minutes to get ready. Yes, it would me too, if someone else had ironed all my clothes, laid them out, got my child ready, organised the event and I had no hair to do.

By the time I got to the Christening I was a sweaty hot mess and forgot the shawl. Nearly sent me under.

I didn't realise baby bag shopping is nearly as important as pram shopping. I loved having my baby bag - along with my baby - with me, but I never seemed to pack the right thing. Those women who carry everything for every occurrence amaze me. Sometimes I'd have three nappies the wrong size and only one baby wipe left. I never achieved the perfect bag, but at least I looked the part.

I had ten months off with Ted and I loved it. I never felt the urge to rush back to work, I didn't miss adult conversation. I was just in Irene and Ted's little world. Unfortunately, we still had to pay the mortgage, so I had to go back. The first day back I was distraught. I was working in Altrincham at the time, a good forty minutes commute, and I asked Adam to bring Ted to work, ready for when I finished at three pm so I could drive home with him. This was a ball-ache trip for Adam, but he did it. When Ted slept all the way home and didn't even notice me I realised I needed to man up and grow some balls.

All that effort and ultimate sacrifice Emily Pankhurst and Emily Davison did for equality and at that time all I wanted was to be a stay at home wife and let Adam bring home the bacon, and I'd make babies and bake cakes … or maybe buy them, the cakes that is.

Three things I am grateful for;

Finally knowing what a mother's love is

Having my mum there to point out the obvious - don't put a rolling baby on a bed.

Big hair

Life is Tough My Darling, But So Are You

My plan was - and you remember how well my plans play out - to have another baby quite quickly. For Ted's 1st birthday we announced I was pregnant again. Now I had conceived once, I was mega fertile. We tried for one month and bam, I was pregnant. I was planning a little girl for Ted to look after. Roll on the twenty weeks scan and it was ANOTHER BOY. I had got quite into Ted and liked having a boy so this time I didn't cry. I resigned myself to living in a house full of underpants, peed on seats and pumping.

Actually, I'll never get used to the pumping part. I really don't know what it is about the male species. Have they got a suction device in their arses which collects air throughout the night, so when they wake up, they cock a leg and fart for England? Is that necessary? Even my ex-husband used to 'fart' in bed and then trap me under the covers. He stopped that when I started crying one day. I even hate the word 'fart'. I'm sure I will continue to have to pull many a finger in a house full of men. Don't get me wrong I do 'pump' I like to call them love puffs, but Adam made me stop staying that. When I was about twelve years old, we were playing out on the street when a police man stopped us to see what we were up to. We all sat on the wall while he took our names -for what I've no idea- when I told him my name I pumped loudly, must have been the nerves. The policeman looked at me and said, 'well I thought you looked like a nice girl' The shame.

I digress, back to making Ted's sibling.

Whilst pregnant with Ted's sibling, we took Ted to the park, it was a glorious sunny day, few and far between in Bolton, and the park was packed. I was sat, or should I say wedged into an elephant on a large spring and Ted came running up to me, he was about 13 months at this stage. He leaned over my lap and I went to pick him up and his eyes had rolled to the back of his head, his body was shaking but his arms were limp. I screamed for Adam whilst running with Ted in my arms. I threw Ted into Adam's arms for him to make it all better.

I turned, like you see on TV, screaming out for a nurse or a Doctor. A lady came running over and stripped Ted off and lay him on the ground. I called for an ambulance. It felt like an age for the ambulance to arrive and by this time, Ted was sitting up dazed and confused. Ted and I had a drive in the ambulance which he was so excited about it. Once at the hospital, the doctors explained it was more likely a febrile convulsion and it was very common in young children. Why did I now know about these things? There weren't in my regular emails about what size he should be, they weren't mentioned in my baby books. This is the kind of shit I needed to know, not he was now the size of a pumpkin seed.

The doctors said to be on the safe side I should get a wee sample from Ted and we should stay in hospital for a couple of hours. Have you ever tried getting a wee sample from a child in a nappy? We took the nappy off and I basically followed Ted's willy around with a cup. I missed. He had another fit soon after, so they were concerned and conducted a lumbar puncture. We were given the choice as to whether we wanted to go in with Ted. I decided to wait outside the room at this point, which in hindsight was not the best as all I could hear was him crying. Everything came back clear so Ted and I just had to stay in hospital overnight to be on the safe side. I slept at the side of Ted in a camp style bed and touched his face all night in case he had another fit. I didn't sleep much. When do you stop worrying about your children? Do you every stop worrying?

This second pregnancy was very difficult, and I was in and out of hospital throughout. I got paranoid about not feeling my second son kick and would sneak off to the hospital during the night while Adam was asleep, get checked out and be back in time for breakfast. I didn't want to appear neurotic - or should I say more neurotic - but things just didn't feel right.

I bled at seven weeks and convinced myself that I had miscarried. I had an early scan and there was his little heartbeat. He was fine. I tried to calm my negative thoughts.

I continued to bleed a lot throughout the pregnancy and my anxiety was through the roof. People told us, 'oh my wife bled all the way through and everything was fine.' I took reassurance in this.

Each milestone we got to, I willed my baby to get to the next one. At our twenty-week scan, the sonographer asked for another sonographer to come into the room and look at our baby, neither of them spoke while they were looking at our baby but then they convinced us he was fine. There was blood within the womb, but they were not overly worried. I felt physically sick and I don't think I breathed while they were both looking. The scan photo we have isn't like a typical scan picture; our baby appeared to be facing the camera looking like he wanted to come out. Adam cried at that photo; our baby wasn't doing too well.

We were told to cancel our family holiday abroad and stay close to home. Although I was desperate for some sun, the thought of going into labour early in a hospital where we didn't speak the language was not appealing. We tried to get a week in Centre Parcs for the half term instead but needed to re-mortgage to afford it. We stayed in the UK for the half term instead and spent far more money than we would have abroad, in shite weather.

Things I am grateful for;

- **Being mega fertile**
- **The NHS for taking care of Ted**
- **Ted's brother for being a fighter**

Dusty Wignall

On 7th November 2013, I had a midwife appointment at 26 weeks and 5 days. I told the nurse I had been having bad stomach pains, she dismissed it and told me it was my stomach growing. I thought it was strange as I had never had this with Ted, and believe me, my stomach had grown a lot.

I'm not sure if it's something that a lot of British people do, but generally when I'm going into an appointment with a doctor I tend to feel like more of a nuisance than someone who's there to get something fixed. I wouldn't say I play down my symptoms, but instead I offer reasons why I'm poorly and pretty much dismiss myself, convincing the doctor I'm not ill in the first place and whatever it is will go away by itself.

I did the same this day and this is something I lived to regret.

I drove home, groaning in pain as I came to each set of traffic lights. A couple of hours later I was on all fours trying to call the hospital. I realised I was in labour - contractions were new to me as I never experienced them with Ted - I phoned the hospital they advised me to have a bath, as they do. The bath did nothing apart from get me wet. I stepped out of the bath and my waters broke all over the bathroom floor. The fluid was full of blood. I shouted Adam and he rang an ambulance. Due to our panic, Ted started crying uncontrollably and could obviously feel our anxiety. My mum rushed round to stay with Ted.

When the paramedics arrived, everything was very subdued. The paramedic went to the bathroom and I know she was looking to see if there was a baby there.

I lay in the ambulance and I just couldn't talk. I'm not a big fan of silence but I just could not speak. Adam made small talk with the paramedics, were they busy, what time they were on till, almost like we were in a taxi on our way for a night out. When we arrived, they checked for a heartbeat and my baby was alive and on his way.

There were lots of people rushing around the room, and an incubator was brought in with a little bag in it which looked like a toasty bag. My little baby would be placed in there to keep him warm and he was probably going to be very poorly. That's fine I can handle that. We can handle that, we are strong. My mum arrived, I had no idea who had Ted now.

My mum came in the room. I looked at her and shouted, 'he's alive mum, he's going to make it'.

About forty mins later they listened to his heartbeat again. The room was ready for him, his toasty bag was ready for him, the midwives - many of them - were ready for him and I was ready for him.

They called for the consultant. The consultant sat at the side of me and turned to a midwife and asked, 'what's her name?' nodding in my direction. I knew then that he was gone. That couldn't be it. Someone do something, get him out and I will do CPR. No one was rushing around. No one was fighting for my baby, only me. It was all a matter of fact. That can't be it.

Dusty Wignall, born 8th November 2013. My second son.

I didn't notice the room clearing but suddenly, his toasty bag was gone, the incubator was gone and most of the midwives were gone. Just leaving two. I remember sobbing like a baby, loud and uncontrollable, I wanted to just curl up in my mum's arms and for her to make it all right again. I know she would have done if she'd have known how. The midwife then explained that I was going to have to give birth to Dusty naturally.

During labour, something I didn't realise, is that the baby helps a great deal with arriving. As Dusty couldn't do this, I had to struggle on my own with the midwives pulling a lot too. I was pushing, this is how I imagined labour to be, but not the part where my baby was lifeless. I was sobbing and pushing, I could see my mum crying into her upper arm hoping I wouldn't see her. Adam was doing what he would have done if Dusty was alive, squeezing my hand, mopping my brow, willing me to push harder, telling me I'm doing great.

Dusty, 2lb 1 ounce, arrived a little bruised but perfect. He was wrapped up and placed in my arms like he would have been had he had been breathing. My tears fell on his gorgeous precious face. Dusty had tiny fingernails and one of his ears had a little imperfection on it just like Ted had had, but that imperfection was perfect. The hospital let us stay in that delivery room all day. We hugged Dusty, kissed him, talked to him, I had a bath while Adam sat in a chair at the side of me, cuddling Dusty and telling him all about how his life would have been in our little family.

Before Dusty was born I was given the option of whether I wanted to see him or not, of course I did, I wanted to inhale every bit of him, so I never ever forgot.

Ten years ago, if someone had told me about a woman who held their baby all day after he had passed away, I'm not sure how I would have felt. It's not until I was in this situation that it seemed the most natural thing in the world.

A photographer came and took some beautiful photos of Dusty and the hospital gave us a little knitted hat to keep his head warm. Obviously keeping his head warm was not imperative but it felt like the right thing to do. We were given a Simba box by the midwife, and it had lots of lovely little things in and little ink pads to get an impression of his feet and hands. They are so special to me now.

Dusty was placed in a little cot. Unlike the normal cots, this cot kept him cold. It had a little plaque on it from another baby that had not made it like Dusty.

Our family came in to see Dusty. My mum and Adam's mum held him, Catherine stroked his little face, Hannah was away at University so couldn't get to see him.

We were with Dusty for around twelve hours. We were still in the delivery room and I know there would have been women waiting for that room so they could have their precious babies, but I couldn't leave that room.

The time came when we had to hand Dusty to the mortician.

The maternity ward is at one end of the hospital and the mortuary was at the other, good planning I guess, one end where you start your life, the other where you end it, with all the bits in between.

This day we walked with Dusty, being held by a young midwife, as that was the procedure, wrapped up in a little blanket with his woolly hat on, through the corridor passing people on the way. Some smiled as we walked towards them with our tiny baby. Their faces changed when they realised all was not right. I couldn't make eye contact with anyone. I held my head low, I was holding it in shame because I couldn't protect my little baby. Our only walk with our son.

The midwife handed me Dusty for one final cuddle and I handed my baby, Dusty, to an older woman dressed in a starch white uniform. I don't remember her face, just that she had mad curly white hair. I had to soak in as much of Dusty as I could as this was the last time I would see him. There is a small bench outside the mortuary where me, Adam and the young midwife sat. I held my head in my hands, Adam has his arm around me, and the young midwife seemed to have an arm round each of us. She didn't cry. Adam and I walked through the hospital numb, watching all the other people going about their own business, passing by pregnant women outside having a quick smoke before their babies arrived. If only they knew what we had just done, would that make them stop? I doubt it. How could they carry on like normal when we had just handed over our beautiful son never to see him again? I remember we didn't speak, just held hands tightly. That night I lay in bed, still with my baby bump, and willed as hard as I could for there to be a baby in there. I held my bump tightly all night and cried myself to sleep.

I had never realised before, bizarrely, is how final death is, that is it; there's no turning back, what if I had done this and that? It was totally out of my control and there was absolutely nothing I could have done to change the outcome. Dusty had done all the hard part by forming all his vital organs, all he had to do was get fat and stay snug inside of me. I struggled with the finality of it all.

When you have a baby the midwife usually comes the next day, I was asked, did I still want a visit? I was annoyed; of course I did, I have had my baby. The next day she didn't come, and I was so upset, how dare they dismiss me just because Dusty hadn't survived? How dare they not recognise his birth? Adam saw my distress and decided to go to the clinic and explain how upset I was and I needed to see a midwife. A midwife came the next day. I loved that he did this for me. It's a bit like me putting maternity pads on his shopping list for him to get. Looking back, I feel so sorry for the midwife who attended. Dishing out the day's appointments that morning, 'right you have go and see Martha and her mummy, you go and see Samuel and his mummy, and you go to see Irene, who's baby didn't make it, plus we forgot to go, so we're a few days late'. I take my hat off to her turning up at my house that day. She arrived, I cried, I shouted, and she just took it. I calmed down.

The next few days came and went, we had to organise Dusty's funeral, that was our focus. I tried to be strong, Judith, my best friend came over with wine and a tiny silver shoe pendant which to this day I have never taken off. We chatted, laughed and drank wine then I just placed my head in my hands and sobbed. Judith is not a hugger and we spent the rest of the evening, hugging and crying. It's strange the things I remember from around that time. My cousin, Maura visited, Dusty shared his birthday with my cousin. On this visit I laughed and chatted like nothing bad had happened, I gave her a birthday card that I had written prior to Dusty arriving and saw her face sadden when she read 'Happy Birthday, love from Irene, Adam, Callum, Ted and Bump.'

The next day, Ted woke up crying for his breakfast. This was normal for Ted, but I couldn't do normality, I had no energy. I picked him up opened the fridge door and said, 'pick what you want, Ted'. This was not the time to be concerned about no sugar, healthy options. I can't even remember what he had, probably a donut, and that was okay, he wouldn't have understood me anyway.

A neighbour knocked on the door. I know that people didn't know what to say, so some people avoided us, which I understand, however, the neighbour stood there with a dish full of shepherd's pie, all she said was, 'put in the oven on two hundred degrees for an hour', smiled and handed me the dish. Small gestures like this will never leave me. I try to do the same myself to others going through hard times, (obviously though I would get them a takeaway or a Marks and Sparks ready meal).

My little sister, Hannah, sent me a Japanese proverb, 'when the Japanese mend broken objects, they fix the damage by filling the cracks with gold. They believe that when something's suffered damage and has a history it becomes more beautiful.' Hannah struggled being far away from me around this time.

My middle little sister, Catherine, brought wine and we cried together.

These aren't massive things, but they are when you are going through the worst time.

I didn't hear from some of my friends, this was hard, but I understood, it became like an elephant in the room when I eventually did see them. With these friends it took a bottle of wine for them to eventually talk about Dusty. But that's all okay.

Our kitchen was full of flowers that had been delivered. From our friends, colleagues, people we didn't know, just to let us know that we were in their thoughts.

We had to go back to the hospital a couple of days later to register Dusty, but as you probably don't know unless you have been in this position, you don't get a birth certificate, you get a still born certificate. Just one breath outside of me, and he could have gotten a birth certificate. I wanted him to have a birth certificate, because he had lived, he had lived in me for nearly seven months. I had felt him kick. He had lived.

I decided to have my hair cut before Dusty's funeral because people said that would make me feel better. That's what women do when they are going through a shit time, a break up, a divorce, having a still born baby? As I sat in the hairdressers with loads of women, some getting their hair cut for a big night out, a hair-cut after splitting with their boyfriends, having spray tans, nails done for the weekend, all I did was put my head in my hands and sob. I wanted to shout out, 'I've just had a baby boy and he is called Dusty'. My second son, I wanted to celebrate him as that's what you did when you had a baby. I wanted to tell everyone how beautiful he was.

The hairdresser owner was Catherine's friend, who I didn't know very well, but she came over to talk about Dusty to me. I admire people like this.

I had never organised a funeral before, I didn't know what to do, and do you send out invites? Is it just me and Adam? What's the protocol for a baby's funeral? I didn't google it this time.

I bought a new black coat and a new dress because that's what I can do, I can spend money. I have never worn them since but still can't bring myself to get rid of them.

We were able to place some things in Dusty's coffin with

him, Ted gave up one his teddy bears and Adam and I wrote a letter, telling him how happy he would have been in our family. I kept his blanket that he was wrapped in and we gave him another blanket, which we had bought for him for his cot. I smelled his blanket every night. That blanket carries so many tears.

The day of Dusty's funeral arrived. I felt strong. Adam had picked the music as that's his thing and something he could do for his son. The two songs he decided on were Berlin Song by Ludovico Eimaudi and I Miss You by The Hours. Six years on and I can only recently listen to these songs without crying. They are beautiful, I would love you to look them up and have a listen and think of Dusty. I decided to buy a set of handkerchiefs for Dusty's funeral. I don't know why but it just felt more respectful. I still have the little blue and white checked handkerchief with my tears for Dusty on it. We arranged for everyone who attended the funeral to wear a blue buttonhole with a little tag with Dusty's name and date of birth on it. I was trying to make as many memories I could in that short space of time.

We waited outside the crematorium and I went and spoke to everyone. I can't remember what I said but probably something like, 'lovely weather isn't it'. The car came around the corner and on the back seat with a seat belt over it, was a tiny white coffin. It looked strange, but cute at the same time. I loved that they were safety conscious with his seatbelt on. My legs weakened, and I felt completely empty inside, I could have dropped to the floor if it hadn't had been for Adam and my mum by my side and my dad's hand on my shoulder.

Death is so final.

Things I am grateful for;

- Having the honour of meeting Dusty Wignall
- Making memories for Dusty.
- Seatbelts

The Difference Between Coping and Healing

The next few days I had now had to contend with physical reminders. I was given a tablet, so I didn't produce breast milk, but they didn't work so now this time round, with no baby to manhandle into a rugby ball position, I had loads of fucking breast milk. Life is so cruel sometimes.

We collected Dusty's ashes in a little purple urn. I told Ted as much as I thought he could handle. We planned to scatter Dusty's ashes at a lovely place near us, where we used to walk and I'd plan our lives - Adam isn't a planner a more let's see what happens, WTAF, so I did the talking. Adam and I went up one evening in December and we had one of those Chinese lanterns. We scattered Dusty's ashes but it was quite windy and the ashes blew back all over us. Then we tried to work the lantern, and this also went to ratshit so, we eventually gave it up as a bad job, not the experience I had planned, it was more stressful than serene.

That night I got very very drunk. I didn't want to feel anything but numbness.

A few months later my mother in law came to see our newly decorated bedroom and Ted found the purple urn and announced this is my baby brother Dusty. We laughed but I could see how this would be a bit awkward. As Callum was a bit older we told him where we had scattered Dusty's ashes on a walk one afternoon. Callum asked if he felt things crunching under his feet would that be Dusty's bones. It's strange the things that make you laugh when you have a broken heart. But you do laugh and it's okay.

I was contacted by a lovely lady from Human Resources

at work, who was probably dreading making the call, she explained that I was still entitled to maternity leave. Trying to see any positives I could, at least I got to spend extra time with Ted and not worry about money. It was hard to enjoy as this should have been time for me, Ted and Dusty together. My auntie told me to always look at things as the first time after Dusty, for example, the first time I took Ted on a walk after Dusty. Once I'd managed a first, the second and third became easier and easier. The first time I took Ted back to a baby class on Dusty's maternity leave, once I had gotten over it, I knew it would be easier each time after that. I tackled everything from this time as a 'First after Dusty'.

I told everyone I could about Dusty which made me feel better but I'm not sure people always appreciated it. Which I can again understand now. I was in Tesco's car park when I saw an old neighbour, she came bounding over, saying, 'you've got two now, what did you have?' She peered into my car to see Ted sat on his lonesome and I told her about Dusty. She looked mortified and it was me that felt sorrier for her.

I am grateful to have got to spend extra time with Ted, but eventually I had to go back to work. Where I work you might not see people for months at a time and I was dreading bumping into people. I got through my first, 'so how's the new baby?' However that question didn't get easier to answer, but thankfully word got around and I wasn't asked too many times.

I was on the phone to a woman from a different office and again I had to explain that Dusty hadn't survived. I told her we had named him Dusty, but it was very clear she wasn't too keen on the name. 'What, Dusty?'

'Yes, he is Dusty Wignall.'
'Oh, right so that's his real name?'

'Erm, yes, it is.' I felt like saying, *how dare you? My baby didn't survive, and you are questioning his name?* But I refrained.

That was it done, surely I'd paid my dues now for my bottle of white musk? But what do I do now? My heart physically ached and I had never experienced anything like it before. I decided to go for counselling. I had to wait till after Christmas for my first appointment. Christmas day was just something I needed to get through for Ted. Ted opened his presents which made me smile watching him. He would have been happy with one present. I walked into the kitchen and cried for my baby Dusty. Adam followed me and just held me. Ted was oblivious, as he should have been.

Waiting for my first counselling session was agony. I had stopped crying. In my head I was thinking, I can do all my crying there and people on the outside will think I'm coping. Keep it together just till you get there. I drove so fast, trying to keep the tears back. I felt like my head was going to explode with tears. I parked my car and could feel the tears starting to roll down my cheeks. Once in the building I had to sign in, it felt like agony holding back, that last five minutes. I got in the room; I can't even remember saying anything, but I must have. I cried for forty-five minutes. The second counselling sessions went pretty much the same way but the third counselling session I felt something very different. Now I'm sure different counsellors work for different people, but this woman, I realised just nodded and didn't speak during the whole time I was there other than say, 'yes, yes,' with a sympathetic face. At this session my crying dried up and

I thought, I'm going to have to punch this woman in the sympathetic face. I refrained, but I couldn't go back.

I got angry with Adam being upset. If I was crying, Adam would hug me, but if he started to cry I stopped, how did he really know? Dusty was my baby and he was in my belly, how could Adam really know this heartache I felt? I know now this was just a stage of grief but I can see how people fall apart at times like this; we don't all grieve the same, there's no protocol as to what to say, how long it will take, what emotion you should feel and when. Thankfully for Adam and I, it made us stronger. It felt - and still feels - like we have this connection between us that no one else can fully understand.

I wanted to make Dusty a positive in my life, not this taboo subject that people didn't mention. I talk about Dusty often, I'll still cry sometimes. My mum said to me, 'you have an allocated number of tears for each of your children and just because he didn't make it doesn't mean you don't still have his quota of tears'.

Around this time, I started to read The Secret. It felt like all my beliefs had gone. I always thought If you tried to live a good ish life nothing bad will happen. Having Dusty left me feeling in limbo. I am a Catholic, but I can't remember the last time I went to church. I am a good person, I try to help others out. I felt like I was looking for answers; an explanation as to why it happened but had no clue where to turn. The Secret felt like it was what I needed at the stage I was in. It did make me question, had I brought this upon myself? Had I convinced myself that things were going to go bad and I put that out to the universe? I'll never know, but I sure as hell was going to try and think good thoughts from now on. I still believe everything happens for a reason, but I have not yet found out that reason for Dusty not surviving. I hate the words died and stillborn, they seem so cold and impersonal.

I like to write down my thoughts, it helps me feel like I am dealing with them, so I decided to contact the head midwife with the following email. Whilst writing the email I felt quite pragmatic about it all. I know that if things had been different and I was treated quicker things would not necessarily have turned out differently. When you're pregnant, whether it be your first or sixth time, you still put your hands and your baby's hands in those of your midwives; they are the experts, they have done this thousands of times before. I felt let down by the midwife I saw on the day at the antenatal appointment and felt she had dismissed me too quickly. I felt let down the day after Dusty was born when no midwife arrived. I didn't want anyone else to go through what I had gone through. I re-read the email hundreds of times before I plucked up the courage to send it.

Dear ****,
I have been passed on your name from the last midwife I saw, *****, from Horwich medical centre.

In November I sadly had a baby boy who was stillborn. I had had a difficult pregnancy with heavy bleeding throughout.

Initially my midwife was ***********, she was lovely. I then had a mix of ****** and another midwife who I now cannot remember her name.

From 20 weeks I was told I had a bleed behind the placenta and needed to monitor my baby's movements and any change, in case I suffered from a placenta abruption.

This was all written in my notes and I told the midwife whom I can't remember her name on my next appointment.

On the 7th Nov I had an appointment with the same midwife but from around midday I started with pains in my stomach. As I was seeing the midwife at 3pm I didn't phone the hospital.

I saw the midwife who said it was probably growing pains. She then asked if I had had an urine sample tested and that an urine infection could be causing the bleeding. I can only assume she either wasn't convinced I had a bleed behind the placenta or she had forgotten and had not read the notes. So I gave her a urine sample.

My pains steadily got worse but due to the midwife saying probably growing pains I put off contacting the hospital. At 6pm my waters broke with a massive amount of blood in them. Once I arrived at the hospital my baby was fine with a strong heartbeat. But I had been in labour and the pains throughout the day were contractions. Forty minutes later when they checked again he no longer had a heartbeat. I then had to give birth to my baby boy, whom we named, Dusty.

I had had an appointment with the consultant who assures me everything that could be done was done, which I have to take her word for. Although she said she was concerned I wasn't told to come to the hospital by my midwife with the pains due to my history and what was in my notes. I have accepted that even if this happened Dusty may still not have survived -this has been hard to accept though-.

I'm not contacting you to apportion any blame but I feel if I had been more assertive with the midwife things would have been different -not necessarily with a different outcome- I also feel I put too much trust in my midwife which I will not make the same mistake of doing if I ever became pregnant again.

I understand she sees many women and I understand now that I should have reminded her each time I had a visit that I had been diagnosed with a bleed behind the placenta, but I was naive in thinking she would remember or read my notes before my appointment.

I have a fourteen month old boy who I had an emergency section with so never had a contraction, if I had have done I would have realised during that day they were the pains I was having.

I want you to be aware of my situation. The midwife was very nice to me and also conducted our antenatal classes with my first baby but I feel very let down by her.

You will probably be aware from ****** that we had to contact the midwifes due to no one coming to see me after giving birth once I was home, which also left me feeling let down again as I had still had a baby and given birth but ***** has apologised for this.

I know I cannot change the outcome of what happened that day but feel it helps me to get through this by informing you of how let down I feel by the midwife and the lack of post-natal contact and just hope this won't happen again to any other person or me in the future.

Kind Regards
Irene Wignall

This was a very hard email to write and, in my head, I thought, that's it, it is done now, time to move on. If only it was that simple.

The midwives did respond and assured me that when or if I got pregnant again this wouldn't happen, and they would make changes so that it didn't happen to other mothers. I just had to take their word for this.

Things I am grateful for;

- **Dusty having a cool name**
- **The Secret**
- **Writing down my thoughts**

Baby Fever

Three months passed and my desire to just have a baby back inside was too much. I had been writing things I was grateful for each day convincing myself and Adam I was okay. We tried again to get pregnant. I believe now that suppressing a sadness like this, manifests later down the line, but I didn't care, I wanted to be pregnant again, I wanted my baby inside me again.

One evening I was in the house alone and I was reading The Secret, with a lamp on. I closed the book and had a strange feeling. I let my head lean back on the sofa and asked myself, was I pregnant? The lamp flickered. This startled me. I turned it off and went to bed with my book. Again, whilst reading all I could think was am I pregnant. The 'big' light startled flickering, I said, is that you Dusty, are you telling me I have a baby in my belly? The hairs on my arms stood on end. I knew it was him. Some people, like Adam, would give me a rational reason for the flickering lights that night, but I knew. The next day I got a test and I was pregnant.

Sadly, I can't remember anything around doing this test. The whole period is very hazy.

This was all I wanted but strangely made me feel so guilty and I felt like I was betraying Dusty. So quite obviously I hadn't dealt with my grief, but I pushed this deep down and pretended. I went to my mum's to tell her and couldn't stop crying, again this was not how it should have been. My pregnancy wasn't enjoyable. I felt guilty for Dusty, as though he may have thought I was replacing him, I felt guilty for my new baby, would he think he was a replacement? I didn't want my new baby to think I only got pregnant again as Dusty hadn't survived. I felt guilty towards my family for what I had already put them through and was now going to put them through, another pregnancy, I couldn't relax, I cried at night in secret. I wanted to fast-forward the forty weeks just to get my baby out. Week twenty scan time. It was A BOY, I didn't expect it to be any different. As long as he survived, I wasn't bothered. I can't remember very much about the pregnancy which saddens me a lot.

What I do remember is being heavily pregnant and shopping in Tesco. Ted had mithered to be in one of the trolleys that had a kid's car underneath. These always seem like a good idea, but they hold sod all of your shopping and are a massive struggle to manoeuvre. I struggled round Tesco, my fat pregnant belly not helping. I got to the check out, sweat running down my face, chatting to the cashier whilst packing my bags, as I turned, I saw a security guard walking in from the car park holding a small boy. I thought, 'aw, he looks like Ted.' I continued to walk out of the store, when I checked in the kid's car I was pushing. No Ted. I ran to the security guard and shouted, 'that's my son!'

He looked at me in disgust and said, 'I have just saved him from running into the car park.'

The store manager came over to see what all the fuss was about, I started crying and protesting, 'I'm a good mum honestly.' There's a bit of a pattern here of me losing children. Whilst pregnant I was closely monitored; I had a scan every two weeks as this is what was promised after I had sent my letter to the head midwife after Dusty. I know the hospital just did this for my benefit and there were no outward signs that this pregnancy was any different to Ted's.

They offered Adam and I some free Hypnobirthing sessions, to calm my anxiety and to get Adam more involved. I am open to trying anything to make a better life, however Adam had some reservations which were confirmed in our first session when we were sat on beanbags and showed a video of a women giving birth in a birthing pool and the partner getting in there with her. I thought it was a lovely image, but Adam couldn't get out of the session quick enough. He is supportive but he has boundaries. The second session we tried some relaxation techniques for when I was in labour. I heard snoring, turned around and Adam was flaked out on his bean bag. Maybe hypnobirthing just wasn't for us.

I was induced at thirty- eight weeks. I had my appointment and walked into the maternity ward with my hospital bag in tow. As I walked in, a midwife greeted me, she explained she was going to be my midwife for the next few hours. She was explaining what would happen, but I never heard a word of it. I will never forget her face, it was the same mid-wife that delivered Dusty. I asked if she remembered me, she didn't. I asked if she remembered Dusty, she did.

She asked if I wanted another midwife, I calmly said no. It was a bond, whether good or bad, but a bond all the same. We both knew Dusty. I wanted her to be with me.

Now, this is a typical mother's guilt. As I cried throughout this pregnancy, Albie Wignall, arrived, crying - after another c section but awake this time. He's now 5 and hasn't really stopped crying, I blame this on myself, as we do. He is healthy, gorgeous, cheeky, very funny and mine, so I'll take the whingeing.

Albie was placed on my chest and immediately went to my boob. This is how it should be. I loved Albie from the minute I placed eyes on him. He looked so much like Ted and Dusty, he was one of us.

Albie didn't leave my side for the first three years, that is unless we were in a car park, at a petrol station or in Next. He decided to do a runner in Next once and headed for the car park outside thinking this was hilarious. I chased after him whilst in the middle of being served at the till and timed the electric doors wrong and hit them head-on, sending me flying back into Next. Albie found this hilarious. I went back to the till after picking myself up off the floor and grabbing Albie. The shop assistant didn't say a word. She knew I was a woman on the edge. If I had had a bottle of wine in my car that day I would have opened it with my teeth and slugged in down in the car. Thankfully I didn't have one.

Things I am grateful for;

- **Albie arriving safely**
- **Normal doors opposed to electronic ones**
- **Not having wine in my car that day.**

You May have to Fight a Battle More than Once

Ted was two when Albie arrived. I had my three boys; two who lived with me and one who lived in heaven. This is what I had decided to tell people if they asked how many children I had, but as time went by I stopped saying this as it made people feel uncomfortable. I suppose looking at it from the other side and someone said that to me I'd think, 'shit. What do I say to that?' It's like when you ask someone are they okay and really you just want them to say yes, not how they are really feeling.

I was supposed to be okay now, I had two healthy sons with me. But I wondered why I felt far from okay.

Ted and Albie look very alike, but personality wise they couldn't be more different. Ted is sensitive, loving, arty and I can see him being a hippy wearing beads around his neck. Albie is the wild one, cheeky but so funny with it, and I can see him wearing a tag around his ankle. However, I am very conscious of labelling your children early on, so Albie if you are reading this later on down the line, by tag I mean, ankle bracelet, not a curfew tag please.

I had another section with Albie but this time I was awake. It was a weird sensation as I could feel something going on with my stomach but thankfully not the pain of it all. As Albie appeared the radio was playing and Candi Statton, You've got the love was playing. We love that song, it's one of 'our' songs. Things were going to be okay. I was so happy that I had Albie safely in my arms but inside I was still so sad.

Albie looked so much like Ted and Dusty. He was perfectly beautiful.

Now I had everything I had ever wanted - albeit not girls. I had my boys, my loving and supportive husband, we both had good careers, nice house, but I was so sad. Even Adam couldn't understand it, and how could I try to explain when I didn't know why I felt this way myself.

I felt like I was acting like a spoilt brat, look at me, how lucky am I to have what I have and I'm still not happy.

I loved Albie as soon I saw him, no getting to know each other, it just clicked. However, I was waiting for something bad to happen to him. It's strange as in my head it was always going to be Albie that something bad would happen to and never Ted. I couldn't explain why I felt this, but I just could not shake it off. Each time he had a temperature I thought calmly, well this is it, this is Albie's time. He once choked in our lounge, he was struggling to cough and breathe, and I sat back for what seemed like an eternity but in all reality was probably five seconds. I had resigned myself to the fact I wasn't going to see Albie grow up. Thankfully my maternal instincts kicked in eventually, and I helped him to stop choking. It was this day I told Adam how I felt. Later I discovered this was me catastrophizing events surrounding Albie, in my irrational state.

Albie was about three weeks old and whilst feeding him one morning around 3am, I got a call from Adam, he was on a night shift at work, 'Don't panic but I'm at the hospital, I've broken my elbow' Don't panic? We have a two-year-old and a three week old, I can't drive for another three weeks, you now can't help with anything neither can you drive, my head is already going to pop off and now you're telling me this. How fucking selfish. 'Yes, babe, I'm not panicking, I hope you're okay.'

We managed, as you do, but it was tough.

A couple of weeks later, Albie had a fever, he had no energy and a rash over his body. I shouted at Adam to get a glass, we pressed the glass against the rash but in all honesty neither of us had a clue what we were supposed to looking at. Around this time, I used to gauge my panic against Adam's, as I knew I was acting irrational and couldn't work out when to worry and when not to. Adam was worried, so I took Albie to A&E. The doctors saw him quickly. It was a brief five minutes of assessment and she told me he was fine and to take him home. They must have seen the worry in my eyes and said, 'if anything changes bring him back'. A couple of hours later I still wasn't happy. I went back. The same doctor on her twenty-three-hour shift came to me. 'Why are you back here?' I couldn't really say because I'm sure my baby is going to die, so I just cried. She sent me home, Albie got better.

When Albie was still just a baby we visited friends for the day. As we arrived Albie shit all up his back. I mean the kind of yellow stuff that covers his entire body. We've all experienced it. My stress levels where quite high and I was taking things out on Adam. On social media I was smashing this motherhood lark but, in reality, my head felt like it was going to implode.

I took Albie straight up to their bathroom to change him and made a right mess and got yellow shit all over our friend's bathmat. I came down to explain, Albie was in a fresh outfit. I held him up and he was sick all over my face and hair. Now normally this kind of thing would make me laugh out loud but, in that moment, I thought, 'this is it, I cannot cope'. I could have placed Albie down, walked away and not come back. My friend, Nic, offered one of her tops but Nic is a gorgeous size 10 and I wasn't anywhere near that. I made Adam take me to the local supermarket to buy me a tent that fit. On our way Adam started to speak and I knew where he was going. I said, 'If you say I have post-natal depression then that's it we are over.' In hindsight even that comment is very irrational but I genuinely meant it.

On the way home, that day I googled post-natal depression and I realised it wasn't wanting to smack your baby's head against a wall as I had thought. I had post-natal depression and to be brutally honest, I was probably still grieving. When I got home, I rang my mum and told her. Her reply was, 'oh I'm so glad you can see it'. I couldn't stop crying, this time with relief. I got help.

Thankfully I had a lovely counsellor this time and I didn't want to punch him in the face.

With Albie I think I took him to one baby massage class, possibly a couple of baby rock and roll classes. I took him to get weighed but on the second occasion when the nurse implied that maybe Albie was a bit fat, I decided to stop going. Looking back now he was enormous so the nurse may have had a point.

On Albie's first birthday, we did what we had done with Ted and he got christened at the same time. I bought a very expensive two-tiered cake, my theme was jungle. You always need a theme. My Pinterest board was full of ideas. The cake arrived in the morning it was amazing. Lions were juggling on the top, I loved it. I went in the kitchen to pay the lady a ridiculous amount of money, that I halved when telling Adam, and Albie walked in behind me seconds later, holding two lions, shouting roar roar. Are you effing kidding me? I ran back into the front room where his lovely two-tiered cake lay on the floor. I turned to the lady, 'Please tell me you have taken a photo?' She couldn't get out of there quick enough. I pieced together the cake and strategically placed it, so it didn't look too bad.

On the day of his actual birthday I bought a £10 cake from Tesco's. We were all sat around singing Happy Birthday when Ted reached in to take a mouthful of the cake, head first, smacked his head on the chair and split his face open. I'm getting the feeling that things are never going to be 'normal' again. Back to A&E.

Before I had children I had a plan of how things would pan out, My GIRLS would be dressed impeccably cute and they'd perform on demand. I now get my kicks dressing them up my boys in outrageous outfits. We love World Book Day in our house and we start planning months in advance. I (and Pinterest) have the ideas, Adam does the putting together.

Me, Ted and Albie - The Stinks as we lovingly refer to them now - became the best of friends. I don't know how I would have coped now with girls, so maybe God's plan was right after all.

Things I am grateful for;

- **Having the Stinks**
- **Getting help for post-natal depression**
- **Not wanting to punch my new counsellor.**

Love is Thicker than Both Blood and Water

As a child I have lovely memories of family holidays, mostly they were in England. We travelled in the summer for two weeks to a caravan park in Torbay. I had new Joe Bloggs jeans and T shirts, I looked the dogs.

The caravan park was spilt into Odds and Evens, Royals and Rebels, and the whole week had all the campers competing against each other to have the most points at the end of each week. My dad entered me into every single activity. Half of which I had never done before. I was in the cross- country race, he ran along the side of the barrier cheering me on the whole way. He entered me into a beauty competition and made me go back to the caravan and change my dress and brush my hair, even allowing me to put on some blue eyeliner and Number 17 lipstick. I was entered the diving competition, albeit I had never stepped foot on a diving board before, suffice to say I never won, but I certainly knew he believed in me. They both did.

When I was seventeen my mum came up to my room, I was sat listening to Sinead O' Connor, nothing compared to you, on my Alba midi hi-fi and said she had something to tell me. This sounds ominous, had she found out I may have tried a splif on Friday night. Oh dear.

She went on to tell me when she met my dad she already had me. Oh no, my mum had lost the plot. I explained that this was not the case as it couldn't have been. My mum had moved over from Ireland when she was eighteen, met my dad and quickly had me, or so I thought. She then explained I was conceived in Ireland by her first boyfriend, nobody in Ireland knew she was pregnant as she wore a corset the whole time, squashing me in -explains a lot, little forehead? At that time in Ireland, unmarried mothers were forced to go to London and give birth to their babies and give them up for adoption a short time later. My mum was petrified this would happen to me and her. She left Ireland. young, pregnant and scared in December 1975 and I was born early February 1976. Mum met my dad a short time later. Wow. I wasn't expecting that. I hugged my Mum. I walked downstairs, my Dad was crying. I hugged my Dad, nothing had changed, if anything I loved them both more. My Mum for being a fighter and my Dad for loving me as much, if not more, than if I was his own flesh and blood.

Three things I am grateful for;

- **My dad for choosing me**
- **My Mum for fighting to keep me**
- **My mum not finding out I had tried a joint**

Excuse the Mess, We're making Memories

Now It was time for Adam and I try to make our own family memories. We decided to book a holiday at Euro Disney when the Stinks were four and two, to make similar memories. The Stinks other brother, Callum, was twelve when we went on this holiday. The car was crammed, and poor Callum was squashed in between two car seats in the back. Once we arrived on French soil Albie started crying and he didn't stop the whole time he was there. We had decided two weeks previously to stop Albie having a dummy. We bought five French dummies on the first day.

We unpacked and then headed out for something to eat. The waitress came to take our order and whilst ordering burger and chips for us all, Albie got hold of the squeezy ketchup and pressed it. Red sauce flew all over my white T shirt and across my face. Oh, how we all laughed. By all, I mean everyone but me.

The holiday comprised of queuing up in the heat for hours on end, Ted and Albie fighting in the confined spaces and then laughing for the thirty seconds we were on the rides. We were queuing for one thirty second ride and Ted got Albie in a headlock and they started to fight, I was sweating trying to pull them apart in the confined space and I clocked another mum looking at me in disgust. How dare she. She was wearing a camping rucksack on her front and a pair of effing Crocs, it should have been me looking at her in disgust ...

We walked back to the hotel, both Stinks crying, Callum wanting to go on the bigger rides with his dad. I turned and looked at Adam, 'what the fuck are we doing?' We decided I would take The Stinks back to the hotel and Adam would take Callum back to park. I asked Adam to get me two double vodkas before he left. He started to moan about the prices in the hotel, then looked at my face. He got me the vodkas.

The one lovely memory was the firework show. We had strategically planned naps and dinner, so we could be all wide awake for the 10.30 show at the end of the day. Callum stood inbetween me and Adam, I was carrying Albie and Ted was in Adam's arms. A spectacular firework shot across the sky and Ted shouted look, 'look, it's baby Dusty'. It made Adam cry. I had no words.

Our drive home from France was long. It was late at night and the motorway was closed so at midnight we were driving through Doncaster trying to get home. Ted wanted a wee. I gave him an empty bottle. He started to wee in it, his willy popped out and he proceeded to wee all over his brothers, the roof of the car and himself. I love my boys…

Ted's wee may have been a premonition as when we walked into the house we discovered there'd been a leak while we were away. Laugh out loud, in a mental rocking in the corner sort of way.

Adam said, 'what are we going to do?'

To which I replied 'We are going to bed Adam. We will deal with it in the morning.'

Our house was in a state of refurbishment for quite a few months, with enormous dryers in every room. Most of our furniture was damaged and had been taken away after being assessed. A lovely well-mannered South African guy came to the house to assess the damage and Albie was pottering around the house. This guy called me Ma'am which I liked. He turned around with his back to me and Albie pressed the Minions fart gun. The man no comment. I think he thought it was me. Me being a Ma'am as well.

Lots of toys were destroyed in the flood and the South African guy took a large bag of them away to be assessed. When I phoned them to see what the damage was, the lady on the phone rhymed off the toys they had taken away: eight Build A Bear costumes, six Batman characters, three Peppa Pig characters, forty-three Happy Meal toys. I started to retort my children don't have McDonalds then I realised I was lying.

The house being empty reminded me of the time we ordered a new sofa from DFS, we had to wait twelve weeks. In my excitement I put our current sofa on eBay for a buy-it-now, well someone did just that, that week, so we spent eleven weeks on bean bags. Oh, how Adam laughed. To give Adam his due he is a patient man. I wanted a new dining table, one day he came home from work to find I had thrown our old one in a back garden and kicked the legs off, so we had to order a new one. Did I say at the beginning of this, I actually became an adult in my thirties? Maybe not.

Adam has always said that when I am my most difficult my boobs have saved our marriage. Who needs Relate when you have big boobs?

Ted is also obsessed with my boobs. As I walk past him he squeezes my boobs like honking a horn. I laughed at first, but when he does it at the school gates I've had to draw the line.

Things I am grateful for;

- House Insurance
- Dusty in the sky
- Big boobs instead of marriage guidance

The Benefit of Being Married to Me is... You're Married to Me

I love buying people presents and I put a lot of thought into them, I'm not sure if it's the giving the gift that excites me or the spending money aspect.

Spending money when I was younger was ace because I had lots of it. I did like credit cards too as that isn't real money. Watching a program one evening about shopping addicts made me stop and think. At the end of the program there was an announcement, 'if you think you have a problem with spending call this hotline.'

Hmmm maybe I do have a little problem looking at all the clothes in my wardrobe still with the tags on. I decided to call the helpline. The phone rang out and then an actual person answered the phone, 'Hello, Shopaholics Helpline.' Shit! I didn't want to actually talk about my problem, I just wanted to leave my address on an answer machine and they'd send me an advice pack then I could feel like I was being an adult about things. I put the phone down on her. Thankfully my spending reduced, partly due to me maxing out my credit cards and partly because now I have no money.

Adam had worked out by now that at birthdays and Christmas, there is a lot riding on what he buys. I love fireworks, but just to clarify I love them on November 5th or at Disney Land. One Christmas before we were married, Adam and I had decided to keep to a fifty-pound budget as we were saving for our new house. I secretly thought he would get me an engagement ring - not out of his budget though.

We sat in bed on Christmas morning, after a lie in, pre-kids, and he handed me a big box. Aw it was one of those jokes, a box within a box within a box and eventually a little ring box. No, it was a box of fireworks. A box of fireworks. I really tried hard to fake it, but I just couldn't. I put the box under the bed and put my thumb back in my mouth and turned over.

Later that same day we went to my mum's for Christmas dinner and my cousin and his girlfriend arrived and announced they had gotten engaged. How sweet, pass me the Baileys; the bottle, not the glass. I couldn't make eye contact with Adam. That Christmas day I finished the night off drunk, falling into the Christmas tree. Why didn't Adam want to marry me?

As you are aware, Adam did get round to proposing to me on Bonfire Night with my nicely timed manicured nails. Adam and I booked our wedding when I was two hours pregnant. I wanted a Christmas wedding. I love Christmas. I love Christmas Eve more; the anticipation. I love the anticipation of every event more than the actual event itself. As planning is my forte, Adam let me plan everything apart from the music. Probably a wise move as the first single I bought was Alice Cooper, Poison,

I loved planning our wedding, funds weren't high as I was on maternity leave, so I had to be strict with my budget. I got a £24.99 wedding ring from Argos in favour of snow globe bride and grooms for the wedding favours. Priorities, I'll get the bling wedding ring later.

I'm still waiting...

I wanted Ted to be involved in the wedding as much as possible. He was five months old when we got married and was able to sit up by himself. That was all I needed for my idea. I was watching two skateboards on eBay and had searched out a wooden crate. I was going to transform these eBay bargains into a Santa's sleigh and I was going to pull Ted down the aisle behind me. Adam said categorically, NO. I was wounded. It would have been perfect. I still think that it was a wasted opportunity.

Due to Ted assisting me lose some of my baby weight by helping me get Sepsis, I was half way to fitting into my dress, but only half way. The pressure I put myself under. I bought my dress when I was three months pregnant, with a plan of only putting on around eighteen pounds, I bought exercise DVDs, 'Exercises to do when Pregnant', joined a gym and did nothing but eat. Resting my Mars Bars on my newly acquired pile of DVDs. I always have the greatest intentions, it's the execution part that I struggle with. My final fitting came, 'it's a bit snug,' the wedding shop attendant said.

'I don't care just get the zip up and I won't breathe, breathing is overrated.'

We got married in front of fifty friends and family. I was surprisingly calm and was able to breathe, a little. I said my vows in a confident voice as I knew how much I meant them, Adam, on the other hand, started crying and didn't stop for two whole days. We were packing the car up the next day with gifts, Ted, my dress, the cake - all into a Vauxhall Corsa - and he started crying, we got home and listened to the play list he'd created for the wedding and he cried again. I am hoping these were happy tears and not, 'Oh my god what have I done' tears.

Three things I'm grateful for:
- **Marrying Adam**
- **Fitting into my dress…just**
- **Having a lovely if not emotional -for Adam- day.**

The Club Scene

Life was ticking along nicely for a while, I had paid my Karma back.

I was back on the slimming club scene. It's the only club scene I do these days. The word diet is now a bad word but, in all honesty, if I can't have what I want, when I want it, I'm sorry but it's a diet.

I have tried them all. When people say I fluctuate between four pounds either side, it really gets my goat as I fluctuate three stone either side. Four pounds, pffft.

I paid £250 to go and sit in a stranger's lounge while he hypnotised me and told me not to eat. I told Adam afterwards, as he would never have agreed to me doing it, obviously knocking the cost down somewhat. He couldn't believe I'd gone to a stranger's house and was willingly hypnotized, I suppose he had a point, anyway it didn't work.

I'm always good for the first three weeks of any diet. I hammer the gym, eat lighter than light mayo and frozen Curly Wurlys. I'd work out my syns/ calories/ points/ pro points to ensure I didn't have to forgo any alcohol. I'd get my half stone certificate quickly; this is the only time I would sit in the class/ meeting/wellness workshop - to get my applause and to tell Gladys how I lost half a stone in three weeks, well, Gladys, I didn't fucking eat. That's the key.

On one of my many inductions I attended a lads' football club meeting room with all the other fat chicks. As I was a new starter, I had to wait till the end to get my 'pack'. There was a few of us new starters this day and at the end of the meeting we all were given our bright green plastic wallets and escorted round the football pitch, through two teams of twenty year old footballers and their supporters, into a separate room. It was like the walk of shame. I bowed my head in humiliation.

But it got worse on the next meeting. I had a 'loss' in my first week so obviously I stayed for the applause. It was the same week the Eurovision song contest was on, so the 'Leader'- to add a bit of excitement into the evening, had created a Eurovision quiz. We all had a partner. I had Shazza, who knew jack shit about Eurovision, like me. We didn't answer one question between us. Then the 'leader' called out the answers for us to mark. Shazza held a pencil against each question number as though she was marking it, I'll give you the heads up Shazza, we have no answers, I'm guessing we will get zero out of twenty. Just a hunch.

The 'excitement' continued and the 'leader' handed out words to a song, about Bran Scran - a piece of cardboard type bread that makes you skinny allegedly pushed by one particular slimming brand - and we had to sing the Bran Scran song to the music of Down Town by Petula Clark.

That was a new low.

I'm slowly learning about body image and being happy with me. We all have our fat photos, ones where we look back now and think, Jeez I wish I was that 'fat' now. I look at social media nowadays and genuinely feel sorry for young girls feeling they must compete with these unrealistic models. Even I follow over forties fashion pages and think, God, how perfect they look.

When I look in a mirror, granted, when I can be arsed putting make up on and brush my hair, I think, 'Hey Irene, you're not looking too bad,' but then I see a photo from the same night and I think, my God, did I really go out looking like that? However, the older I get, the more I don't give a toss what people think of me. If I feel good and Adam still fancies me, that's good enough for me.

Things I am grateful for;

Being part of a club scene
Frozen Curly Wurlys
Acceptance

In My Line of Duty

I am a Detective in the police and have been in the police for 20 years. I am fortunate to have had a very varied career. Being a police officer is sometimes stressful, emotional, shocking but most of all you feel like you have a second family; people you trust and who have got your back.

When I was younger the police, were feared but these days no one gives a toss. Partly due to the lack of police officers and I'm not naive in thinking all police officers are good - you have bad eggs in every job and nowadays, there's generally a lack of respect around - wow, how old do I sound?

When I was about eleven my friends and I decided to bring our felt tips out and graffiti on the pavilion on the football fields near our houses. I wrote things like 'Irene woz ere', because that sentence sounds so cool. A policeman saw the graffiti and found us, surprising, as he was probably looking from an escapee from an old people's home after reading my graffiti. He made us all go home and get dishcloths and wipe it off. That pavilion had never been as clean. We bricked it. I was so good the next few weeks trying to gauge if the police had contacted my mum and dad and tell them they had raised a criminal. On a positive note I never pumped in front of this policeman.

I never put this on my police application form.

Being in Police along with feeling that you are a making a positive difference to people's lives, there were also other perks to the job.

One-night shift I was called to a stabbing in the city centre. I got there, and uniformed officers were already there with the paramedics, one rather good-looking paramedic too, I noticed from the corner of my eye, whilst I was getting all the details of which hospital the victim was going to. The ambulance left the scene and I spoke to the uniformed officers. I might have happened to mention in passing that one of the paramedics was a bit fit. In the early hours, the uniformed officers came back from speaking to the victim and handed me a number. 'That's the paramedic's number for you.' OMG, how desperate must I have looked? I said, 'thanks' and quickly put the number in my phone.

Later that day I spoke with the Paramedic and discovered we lived in the same town. Not only that but he lived on the same street as a girl I car shared with, so we arranged to go on a date the next week. We continued to text throughout the week, then the day before our date I was collecting my friend from the same street to go to work. He had just finished nights and told me he'd look out for me. As I drove around the corner, I saw an image of a bloke in a green uniform, as I got closer, I realised this was not the paramedic that I had liked on the night of the stabbing, but his van partner. And I know this sounds very very shallow, but I did not fancy him at all. I waved as I drove off with gritted teeth saying, 'oh shit what have I done?'

He texted me later in the day asking if our date was still on. Dilemma. What do I do? Cruelly dump him after seeing him, or go out and end up probably kissing him out of sympathy? So, I cruelly dumped him. I didn't have another date for about 12 months after that, Karma for being so shallow.

I'm not going against National Security here as everyone knows the police sometimes conduct surveillance. One of my jobs required me to go and do a recce with a colleague in plain clothes. We were in a high sided van. I was nervous as this was my first time doing anything like this, I had to prove to myself and my colleagues that I was up to the task.

As we were driving to the location I was going through my cover stories; what I would answer if I was asked any questions. We pulled up at the desired location, 'nice and discrete now Irene', my colleague reiterated, 'nice and discrete.' 'Yes, yes I've got it'. I took my seat belt off, adrenaline pumping through my veins, heart pounding. I opened the van door, forgot I was in a high sided van and stepped out. I fell like a sack of shit on the pavement. I've never jumped us as fast in my life. Nice one, Irene, nice and discrete.

Apart from this, I am good at my job and can deal with people from all walks of life. However, I take my hat off to anyone who works with old people, I just cannot do it without crying. Once, we had a report of a missing old women who had dementia. A few hours later she walked into a community centre telling them that her husband mentally abuses her. We went and spoke to the lady and realised that the person she was talking about was her first husband from thirty years ago, her now husband who was frantically looking for her was not the abuser. I went to get him, he was so worried and relived she was safe. He got some wedding photos out to remind her. We walked into the room she was in, I said, 'look who I've brought to see you, it's your husband'.

She took one look at him and shouted, 'that's not my husband'. I burst into tears seeing the man's heartbroken face and had to leave the room. I needed to get out of the building, but all the bloody doors had security locks on them, so the old people don't do a runner. That day the catering staff saw a crying Detective running through the kitchen while they were making toad in the hole. I had to take three hours annual leave that day as I just could not stop crying. I drove straight to my mum and dad's house and immediately on opening the door started to cry again. My mum and dad thought the worse, maybe I had seen a murder victim, a rape victim, a serious road traffic accident. No, it was a little old woman who didn't recognise her husband. It was at times like this I thought I was maybe in the wrong job.

Three things I am grateful for;

- The man who was stabbed made a full recovery
- I don't work with old people all the time
- I always check what kind of vehicle I'm sat in before getting out.

This Time Next Year, Rodders

I'm a bit of a Del-boy at heart. I have thought of every and any business I could do rather than working for someone else. I made birthday cards, they looked like Ted had made them. I made Tutus, they were pretty, but Ted and Albie started to refuse to try them on for me after a while. I created my business name 'WigglyBones'. I loved it. I loved it that much I registered it as a trade mark. I even bought a private registration plate saying Wiggly. Remember that name, as one day it will be famous. It must be as I paid £200 for it to be registered. I'm just not sure what it will be famous for yet? Minor details.

I made memory jars and even contacted companies in Taiwan, knowing nothing about exporting. I still get emails from them addressed Dear Wiggly. I wonder if they really think that's my name.

I enquired about opening a soft play franchise. It was only £75,000, a bargain. Adam just rolled his eyes. He tended to do this a lot when I had an amazing business idea to put to him.

I bought forty-five pairs of elf slippers from a company online that dealt in bankruptcy stock. Adam said the clue was in the title. I ended up giving the last ten pairs to charity. I have visions of ten kids from Ethiopia, well chuffed walking their three miles, to and from school in Elf slippers.

I tried network marketing. I think most people in their lives have tried some sort of network marketing, I remember as a kid, women used to go to Tuppawear parties, then there were Anne Summers parties. Some people bought loads of Hoovers and went door to door to sell this revolutionary Hoover. I wonder if Richard Branson ever tried network marketing?

When I decided to give it a go I think everyone else decided to give it go at the same time. I convinced myself that Aloe Vera was the future. I even had a team and we waved team flags at events. We had team meetings at my house, my dining table was now my boardroom. This was it, this was my turning point, I really believed it. I threw out all the products we had already and bought Aloe Vera products, much to Adam's exasperation. I had to, I needed to earn my commission. I convinced my family to do the same. I spent money left, right and centre. It was fine, I was going to earn it all back anyway. I hired stalls at local fairs, the only people who came to speak to me, were themselves part of the Aloe Vera tribe or weirdos who just wanted to talk to someone. I quickly realised Aloe Vera was also everybody else's turning point too and the market was flooded with Aloe Vera sellers. I say, quickly realised, it took me eighteen months to see.

Even though Aloe Vera was not the one for me, it did prove to me that I could do something more than just being a Police Officer. I even spoke in a room full of fellow Aloe Vera-ers and told them how successful I was becoming and going to be and how it was the business for them, as I truly believed it at the time. Public speaking had never been for me but I did love the buzz as long as I had a glass of water for my dry mouth as my lips slowly curled up mid-speech.

I played with writing a blog and decided to put myself out there on Instagram. I am old school. I have a love/hate relationship with Facebook but had never tried Instagram. So, my first time and this is what I encounter. This is normal right? So, I get my first Instagram message after my first attempt at a blog, probably talking about my lack of control of The Stinks. It's from a lovely girl who says she's enjoyed reading my blog and makes small talk. I oblige as I think this is all okay. She then asked for a photo of me? Normal right? As I'm new to Instagram I struggle to send a photo, so she says, 'its fine here's my number, WhatsApp me it's nice to put a name to the face'. This sounds acceptable but naive maybe - I'm a cop for God's sake - I send a WhatsApp and the conversation continued there. I get slightly paranoid when she compliments me repeatedly, so I slip in the fact that I'm married, and all is great. She sends me photos of her and her husband. Phew, I was barking up the wrong tree, this girl just wanted to be friends.

Then I get a message saying her and her husband like to spice things up and she likes girls and she likes me. I knew it I wasn't being paranoid. I explain the messages to Adam and show him and he comments that I have been flirting with her. Oh my God, I was just trying to be friendly back but yes, re-reading my messages, she says my hair is nice and I reply, so is yours.. Her hair is quite funky, so I say, it's good to be different. WTF, had I lead her on? The messages go on mostly on her part and in the end, I return to Google.

'How do you block someone on Instagram.'

Delete. Lesson learnt. About six months later I get a friend request on my faithful Facebook from her husband. Seriously I don't think I'm ugly but in the big world wide web there are far, far prettier people out there.

I'm too old for this shit.

Apart from being propositioned for a threesome I did enjoy writing my blog, I was very average in English lessons at school and can't ever remember as a child, reading books, although I'm sure I did. I started writing more and more and discovered if I got my thoughts out on paper it somehow organized my mind. I have always had lots going on in there.

It became a focus of mine, empty my head a couple of times a month on paper and make some order inside my mind.
 I knew in my heart I had something else to give but just as I was getting some order, I had to put it all on hold as I was about to encounter another of life's challenges

Three things I am grateful for;

knowing where I am with Facebook

doing my first public speaking even with curling lips

my friends not disowning me during my Aloe Vera phase

The life of Brian

About two years ago I started being very tired and I thought it was just family life and it was how everyone felt. I went to the doctors for blood tests, everything came back fine. I went once to see the nurse with Albie in tow and she greeted me with, 'Hello lovely to meet you and this must be your grandson?' She saw the look on my face and went on to say, 'I would have got it wrong no matter what I said'. Excuse me, no, you would have got it right if you had said, 'is this your son?' I would have started with that if I were you, you muppet. Note to self – make an appointment for Botox.

So it was confirmed I was just extremely lazy and couldn't hack bringing up a family, working and all that came with those things, let's not forget old looking.

I also started to feel dizzy a few times at work, nothing to write home about just the odd off balance which I put down to drinking on a school night. I convinced myself I just needed glasses, so I booked an eye test. Whilst waiting in the shop, I picked the glasses that made me look most intelligence. I tried on a lot … I went for the test and my eye sight was perfect.

The optician advised that I went for a hearing test. I got an appointment that same day and had a hearing test with what looked like a fifteen-year-old lad in a suit that was too big. He went on to tell me my hearing was not where it should be for my age. He was very careful with his words, but he managed to imply that due to my age I would be going a bit deaf anyway. I hate these reality-checks to my age. He gave me a form to give to my doctor. I have since been back to thank this teenager as he probably saved my life. He was on honeymoon when I went back so I might have exaggerated slightly about him being fifteen years old. I saw the doctor a couple of days later, a student doctor, again fifteen years old-ish. She looked at the form and asked me 'Okay what would you like to happen next?' Eh?

I was referred, thankfully, and within a couple of weeks I was having a MRI scan. I have been through a lot and consider myself strong but things like this make me want to cry. I know kids have these scans so that stopped me from crying. I tried not to worry too much about the results, but bizarrely hoping that there was something wrong otherwise I was just a lazy woman going a little bit mad.

I was told I would get the results back within three weeks. Three days later I received a letter with an appointment to go and see the consultant for the following Wednesday. This felt too quick. The NHS wasn't this efficient if there was nothing wrong. I had to sit down when I read it because I knew it wasn't good news. My family said, 'it will be fine', but I know we all thought the same thing. When we talked about what it might be we spoke in a jolly upbeat way like it was going to nothing really. I'd already had some tests which confirmed my balance. These tests were very surreal. I had goggles on and had to follow a light spot on the wall, at the same time as doing this they shot air and water down each ear to see how my eyes coped. Who thinks these things up? It was confirmed my balance was deteriorating on my left side and I was referred for physiotherapy. It wasn't a hangover. Phew. Carry on with the wine. So far, I've had physio for breathing and now physio for my head to stay balanced. Wow, who knew?

At one of my appointments for physio I was sitting in the Audiology Department waiting room. There was just me and a sweet-looking very old woman. The nurse came out and said 'Hilda?' Now I know I have an old-fashioned name, but looking at me and the old women, if I was the nurse I would have made an educated guess as to who Hilda was. Me and Hilda both stared forward. Again, the nurse said, 'Hilda'? Hilda then looked at the nurse and said, 'Sorry are you saying something, I'm a bit deaf'. No shit, Sherlock, sat in the audiology department. I'm no expert but maybe a sign with your name on would be more beneficial in a waiting room full of deaf people?

My physio was strange; it was just a case of my standing on one leg, marching on the spot with my eyes closed and discovering I'd travelled to the other side of the room, or , looking at a 'X' written on a post it note and shaking my head. Bizarre.

The day of my appointment to see the consultant arrived, Adam came with me. I could have cried in the waiting the room, anxiety was literally beating out of my chest. I had to concentrate on breathing, thinking, 'please don't forget how to breathe again. I have enough going on.' I expected the consultant to say, 'Hello, Irene', and I would burst out crying, snotting all over him. Thankfully that didn't happen. I kept the snot and crying contained till I left that appointment.

Sometimes little things happen around you; little signs that everything is not okay if you're watching closely enough to notice. I love people watching. The little sign for me then was that when I was called in for this appointment a nurse came in too. Whilst watching all the other appointments she never went in with them. The consultant was lovely and knew my name, a positive from my experience. He then stated.....'It's nothing sinister but you have a brain tumour.'

Shit. I have no life insurance. In fact the application form was in my car all filled in, in a self-addressed envelope, waiting to be posted and had been for about a month.

I focused on all the negatives that came out of his mouth. Thankfully Adam focused on all the positives. He went to explain it was benign - which, apparently, he could tell by looking at it - and what would happen was that I would get referred to Salford Royal Hospital to see the experts in this kind of thing. I couldn't think of anything to ask him at the end of the appointment, so we shook hands and left. In the corridor Adam hugged me hard. If this was God's pay back for me stealing a bottle of white musk from The Body Shop when I was fourteen years old, it was a bit harsh. I bloody wish I'd stolen the Dewberry as well.

We hugged in the corridor, Adam was trying to say all the right things, 'the consultant said it wasn't sinister. It will be okay, we've come through other things. You're strong'. But that's the thing, I didn't want to have to be strong again, I was done with that. I had already proven myself, why oh why did I have to prove myself again? I was happy plodding on with life and my major drama being Albie doing a runner in a shopping centre. Why couldn't someone who had not lost a baby have this tumour? I wanted to have a tantrum, stamp my feet and shout out, 'it is not fair', but life isn't fair sometimes.

Adam went on to reassure me that everything would be okay, but this is what he said when I was freaking out when I was pregnant with Dusty and everything did not turn out okay, so I struggled to accept what he was saying.

I don't know how long I had had this tumour, it could have been in my brain from birth, or it could have arrived after

Dusty, I will never know. In my heart, I think it arrived after Dusty, after I tried to supress all my sadness, but I will never know for sure. But as the saying goes you never know what worse luck your bad luck has saved you from. So, it could have been worse, I guess.

I was told to go home and try not to think about it as I had to wait six months to see if the tumour was growing.

We came home to my mum and dad's house as they had Ted and Albie. I sat on the couch in my mum's front room and explained what the consultant had said, my voice going higher at the end of each sentence. Ted and Albie were jumping on my head as was the norm. My mum walked into the kitchen on her own, I knew she wouldn't cry at this moment because my mum's priority is us girls always; she would be strong for me. Dad cried, which I expected, as my dad cries, that's his thing. He cried at Dallas when Bobby died. He cried at The Waltons, and I've even seen him cry at Neighbours when Mrs Mangle died. I felt guilty that I was making my mum and dad sad again, they deserved a break from shite too. We had decided to go out for tea regardless of the outcome. I was trying to be all positive and so was my mum; that's what we do. I was explaining that this was the best brain tumour that I could have as brain tumours go. Lucky me.

We ordered our food and an unimaginable thing happened, I had lost my appetite. Thank you, God. Unfortunately, I hadn't lost my lust for wine and I had about 1000 calories worth. What he gives with one hand he taketh away with the other.

Things I am grateful for;

- Having 'the best' tumour
- Losing my appetite
- Being saved from the worse luck with just having bad luck

When you're Grateful for Bare Arses

Trying not to think about a brain tumour which may or may not be growing in your head is a bit difficult. It was the last thing I thought about before I went to sleep and the first thing I thought about when I opened my eyes. That is unless there was a bare arse in my face. Not Adam's. Ted and Albie would often strip off during the night and end up in bed with us, so I was quite grateful for the days I was woken up by bare arses as those were the morning I didn't think tumour.

I love how in times like this you can come down to reality with a bang. I had a week off work when I was first diagnosed. To spend some time with my family, get things straight in my head and wallow in some self-pity and wine which thankfully was allowed.

One early morning I went downstairs and both boys were fixed to the TV watching Scooby Doo. You must have watched Scooby Doo regardless of what age you are and seriously, it's just the same story repeatedly, the Pesky kids solve the mystery. This time, Ted had asked me for a drink, there was a cup on the dining table full, so I said, 'well who's drink is this?' No reply. I often speak to myself. I took the drink and had a mouthful. Ugh, it was warm. 'Albie', I asked, 'have you filled this with warm water'? As it is usually Albie.

Albie decided to listen this time and replied nonchalantly, 'No I've wee'd in it'. Are you effin serious? I gagged on the thought of the big mouthful that I had just swallowed. Boom, back to reality.

I started to tell people about the tumour, whose official title was an Acoustic Neuroma Schwannoma, I tried to do it in a jolly way, 'hi, how are you? Yes fine, how's the kids. Nightmare as always. Got a bit of a brain tumour going on, but we've booked a holiday. Are you going away?' It was like a conversation in a hairdresser, with the talk of a brain tumour just slipped in there. It's amazing how many people go on to tell you, 'oh I h've had a friend of a friend who had a tumour'. Jesus, let me just have my moment. It's times like this you can be selfish. I didn't want to hear, 'well at least it's not cancerous'. Well, do you effing want it then?

I had a conversation at The Stinks swimming lesson with a dad. He had heard about my tumour and went on to tell me how his uncle had one three years ago. He had the operation to remove it.

'Oh, so how is he now?'
He died.'
Ah alright, cheers for that.
I know people just don't know what to say and I'm sure I have been the same in the past, but I'd like to think now the shoe has been on the other foot I would say something different.

I phoned Catherine and Hannah and let them know. Hannah was devastated she was so far away - she was brave enough to move more than fifteen minutes away from our mum and now lives in London. Catherine came around with wine. We got drunk and Christened the tumour Brian.

On the outside I was coping, I laughed it off like a zit on my chin, but I was angry, really fucking angry that I had to be strong again, strong for my family, strong for Ted and Albie who expected nothing less, nor should they.

I had to wait for a six-month gap between my two scans to see if the tumour was growing. In the meantime, I sent the forms off for life insurance. Shockingly, I was rejected. Arseholes.

We decided we needed a holiday in the sun but as we had now learnt from our Disney holiday we agreed it was better to have an increase in the adults versus child ratio. My mum and dad came along as well as Adam's mum. It was going to be cosy, us all sharing a villa, but it could work.

We arrived at our villa and it was perfect; a brilliant pool for the kids and lots of outdoor space. We made lunch and the lads quickly got their trunks on and inflated their lollipop floats. Ted had had swimming lessons since he was ten weeks old. Albie joined me on Ted's lessons as he was just a baby.

As Ted was two I had to get in the pool with him and I put Albie in an orange baby float. I'd be concentrating on Ted when I'd look around for Albie. He would be at the other end of the pool bobbling along having no idea where he was, usually asleep. On our holiday they both were okay swimmers but as a precaution I bought a life vest for Albie, from Amazon. He was fuming when it arrived, it was pink, but I managed to convince him it was a shade of purple.

They eagerly got in the pool and I put my lovely new holiday dress on for lunch. It was going to be very civilised, eating in the dining area, overlooking the pool with a glass of wine in hand. As we were all chatting, and the lads played, I glanced around to see Albie under the water, a pink life vest strewn on the side and Ted trying to save him, I jumped in with a mouth full of crusty bread and my new dress on. Fifteen minutes we had been there, and I had already saved my drowning child. Hmmm, maybe this wasn't going to be the relaxing holiday I had envisaged.

Albie got his revenge on me for the pink life vest on one of the nights I put them safely to bed and went downstairs to enjoy the wine. Around an hour later, we all decided to go to bed and I checked on the lads, Ted snoring away, Albie, not in his bed. I checked all around the room, trying not to panic. No signs. I alerted Adam, we started frantically running around the villa, all I could think about was Madeline McCann. I ran out into the street, no one was about. We had earlier covered the pool as we did in an evening, I looked at the cover and thought, oh my God, what if he is under there? Adam then shouted from inside, he had found Albie hidden under our bed fast asleep. Deja vu? In the morning he thought this was a hilarious trick he'd played on Mummy and Daddy. Yes, Albie effing hilarious.

After our holiday I had thought I would have felt rejuvenated and raring to tackle the next stage head on (literally), but it had the opposite effect. I dropped The Stinks off to school a couple of days after we got back and was due in work at eleven o'clock. All I had to do was go home and pick an outfit to wear for work. As I was driving back home this tiny task enveloped my head and became insurmountable. I couldn't cope. I couldn't deal with Brian the Tumour, being a mum, being a wife, being tired all the time, being a detective and now on top of all that, picking an outfit, all at the same time, something had to give, or I was going to lose the plot. I phoned in sick that day and straight away I felt like a massive weight had been lifted from my shoulders. My priority now had to be me.

Now having the worry of work removed, I started meditating, Thai Chi, writing down my thoughts again and healthy eating - that last one is a lie. I continued to write down three things I was grateful for each day. Some would be poignant, most would be mediocre. For example, Albie went to bed and only got up five times before he went to sleep, but it meant that I was focusing on positive things and that's the main thing. That's when I started to write this. I always had a diary as a kid and still have them in the attic now. I cringe if I read them now. You think you have issues as a thirteen-year-old but being grown up is hard. The highlights of my teenager diaries were top ten boys in my form and marks out of ten - this changed often as I was/am very fickle, details about drinking a can of Stella and my boyfriend being sick and wanting to kiss me afterwards, and not having anything short to wear for the school disco that was held in a convent. First world issues.

Post-holiday my appointment came to have the second scan and this time I was told I was going to be injected with dye to get a clearer picture of the tumour. I lay down absolutely shitting getting an injection in my head when she came along and put a tourniquet on my arm and injected the dye there. Phew. I really did think she was going to stick the needle in my head.

I had lots going on in my head, part of me wanted the tumour to be growing so I could have the operation to get it out. If it wasn't growing, I would be scanned every year and the waiting and not knowing each year seemed worse than having surgery to me. I wanted it out, so I could crack on with the rest of my life and stop having to 'be strong' as this was just a major inconvenience. Things I am grateful for;

Things I am grateful for;
- **Not being injected in my head**
- **Haven't drank wee since**
- **Learning how to spell tourniquet.**

Mummy Juice

After phoning in sick, I knew I had to focus on my wellbeing. I did another lot of finding myself, soul searching, sorting out my once again fucked-up head, call it what you want. My wellbeing should be a priority not something I put off till I get more time, money etc. It's funny as it takes something drastic for me to start thinking about my wellbeing again. And the thing I have realised about wellbeing is it needs to be a long-term life choice not just something you delve into when you are going though difficulties. A bit like how I should treat a diet I've been told, not just a quick three weeks here and there.

It's around this time I dabble with being teetotal. I know, I can't believe it myself. I've joined another club, this time called One Year No Beer. I'm enjoying this club. I've always had a love-hate relationship with alcohol. I love it, it hates me. It was all fun and games when I was younger, drinking strawberry Mad Dog 20/20 in the park in my teens, moving onto to sambuca and cheeky Vimto's in my twenty's. Then onto wine and vodka, (not together), in my thirties. Adam doesn't particularly drink; he'll have a couple of pints if he's in the mood, but he never drinks in the house. This felt like a challenge for me at first. I'll get him up to my level. He could go to gigs and drink pop. I'd never met anyone like him. Weirdo. After a month of being together he said his alcohol intake had tripled. My mum advised me this wasn't something to be proud of, but secretly I was.

After the first couple of loved up months, he went back to drinking pop. I learnt to love this as I always had a taxi. We had a rule - if we went out with my friends, he would drive and if we went out with his friends, I would pay for the taxi. I didn't do going out and not drinking. I just couldn't see the point. Neither could I see the point in just having one.

I would have a glass/bottle of wine after a hard day, after a good day, celebrating, commiserating, any reason really. Everywhere I looked it seemed to validate drinking as being a mum was hard work and everyone needed wine to get through it. Don't get me wrong, I wasn't drinking wine for my breakfast, in Wetherspoons at 10am or carrying it in a brown paper bag, but slowly I started to think that maybe it just wasn't worth the foggy next days and watching Adam enjoy things probably more than I did whilst he was sober.

All this made me start to question my reason for drinking. But I questioned it whilst still drinking for about two more years, so it wasn't a rushed overnight decision, I had thought long and hard about it over a glass of wine or three. I realised I had got into a very bad habit that was a struggle to get out of. Some would call that dependent, but presently that's too strong a word for me. I like to use the term that I was an irresponsible drinker. I had no cut-off point and for many years this didn't bother me. It was all part of the going-out process, speaking the next day and discussing what I did as I couldn't remember. Oh God, I didn't tell my auntie she had a haircut like a Lego head did I? It was all part of the ritual, part of the fun … for a while.

I know, I'll give up the wine and get hooked onto exercise instead. I'm still waiting for that last part to kick in.

I'm not going to bleat on about how alcohol is a toxin blah, blah, blah, I've had Botox for God's sake, but I do think it's worth a dabble at being teetotal if it's on your mind. It's now fashionable to be, 'Sober Curious'. Life doesn't suddenly become great and you are able to run marathons, but it does give you a strange clarity. I'm not sure how I would have coped with losing Dusty without wine. I would have coped, because we do, but I probably would have 'felt' more and I didn't want to 'feel' at that time I wanted the numbness that wine gave me.

I don't regret my relationship with wine, I had some amazing nights with it, but I had also had the beer fear, overdosing on carbs the next day, beer goggles, anxiety, the checking Facebook in the morning worried what I would find on my profile. Thank God social media wasn't around in my twenties. But I was now thinking could I have had those amazing nights without the alcohol?

I used to think people who didn't drink were a bit odd. My Irish grandfather used to say don't trust a man who doesn't drink. But now I'm one of them, well I am a bit odd so maybe he was right.

I have completed dry January before, well twenty-eight days of it, but I will take that. I knew I wanted to stop drinking for my health this time. Having a brain tumour was serious shit and after my battle to get my little family, I didn't want to piss it up the wall so to speak. If you stood The Stinks next to a glass of wine and said which would you pick to have forever there would be no competition, it would be the wine. Just kidding. I know this sounds dramatic, but this is how I felt.

If my tumour was growing then my head was going to be cut open and people were going to be poking around in my brain, I wanted my brain to have a fighting chance and not be pickled in vodka when they peeled back the layers.

Also, a big deciding factor was The Stinks now called wine,

mummy juice.

I look at The Stinks and I want them to experience everything they can in life, going to a gig, their first holidays, getting their first girlfriends/partners. But I wanted them to really experience these events, whilst not having the mask of alcohol to numb any feelings. I wanted them to live life and then decide if they would like to drink alcohol.

I read lots of books about quitting alcohol - in the 'club' it's called quit lit - my first one and most impressionable one was This Naked Mind by Annie Grace. I say I read it but I haven't got the patience to read so I listen to the audio books. Annie Grace's voice is amazing. She sounds so super cool, so if someone super cool can give up the alcohol then surely, I could. I've listened to this book three times and will probably listen again in the future. If one of my dreams has come true and you are listening to this on audiobook then my voice has a broad Boltonian accent, with a slight lisp through forty-three years of sucking my thumb, so I may ask Annie to read this instead.

It was nice as well, when a consultant asked how many units of alcohol I drank a week not to have to lie, now I could say zero and make eye contact at the same time.

I stopped drinking alcohol December 31st, 2018 at 10pm.

Three things I am grateful for;

🌀 **Quitting alcohol**
🌀 **Finally feeling things**
🌀 **Having Wine in my life when I lost Dusty**

The life of Brian (continued)

After a lot of chasing up I finally got my result. Brian, was growing. It seemed bitter-sweet. After I left the hospital, I bumped to one of my auntie's friends, Brenda. Brenda was having a lovely day shopping with her daughter when she asked me, 'you alright kid?' This was one of those moments when I should have said 'Yes, you?' But I started to cry and blubbered to her in the middle of the street, I made her cry. Her daughter didn't have a clue what was going on, then I rushed off.

Now I had to think about surgery. There was a waiting list of twelve weeks so that was the end of February. As they were going to shave some of my hair, I decided to cut it short anyway and style it out. Brain surgery is no excuse for bad hair. I had a series of injections in my ear to take away my balance which was very unpleasant. These were one a week for three weeks. The first was uncomfortable but I got through it. With the second and third as I knew what to expect, it became harder and I was pulling away when he went to inject me. It was like I had no control over my head.

My first appointment at Salford Royal was with a very handsome consultant. The type that you see on the TV: smartly dressed but with his skirt sleeves rolled up like he had just rushed out of surgery having saved someone's life. Adam was with me, so I kept that thought to myself.

The handsome consultant wanted to see the movement in my face and asked me to frown and smile, show him my teeth etc. I couldn't for shame tell him - or Adam for that matter - that I had Botox two weeks previously and if anything was moving I was going to get my money back. I also had new teeth in ...

I am a marketing person's dream customer, adverts were made for people like me. I watch something and immediately cannot comprehend how I have gotten through life without said item and I need to buy it this minute. Internet shopping created a whole new level for me. I could order things and they would arrive the next day before I even had to think about if I really needed the item or if I could even afford it.

These days I'm trying to use the 'magic twenty' rule - before I make any hasty purchases I think of twenty reasons for and against why I should buy the item. I forgot to do this before I ordered the new teeth off the internet. There's nothing particularly wrong with my teeth, they're just little and I always wanted big teeth. Well, when they arrived, they were big! Adam took the piss out of me when I tried them on, another £360 down the drain. But for some reason I had decided to wear them this day.

I'm sure the consultant could tell, partly because he was blinded by the whiteness.

I had a further appointment a few weeks later to go through the risks with the two consultants who were going to be doing the surgery. I didn't wear my new teeth this time. Call me shallow, but one of the risks I was dreading was my facial nerve being damaged. I didn't want to scare The Stinks and I didn't want Adam to just love me; I wanted him to always fancy me. The appointment to go through the risks was a bit too long for my liking. I had been working on my wellbeing trying to focus on the positives and now I had to sign a form full of negatives;

- Facial nerve damage
- Higher risk of a stroke
- Dry eye, eye lid dropping

- Brain fluid leakage

The jolly list went on.

I was informed that the surgeons would take a piece of my skull away and rather than put it back they would take fat from my stomach and use that to fill the hole instead. It seemed a bit odd to me, but hey, I'm not stopping anyone taking fat from my stomach. I thought I was funny when I said, 'oh, you can take as much as you want'. I bet the surgeon had only heard that comment hundreds of times. He tried to feign a smile.

I had explained to Ted and Albie that I had a 'spot' on my brain and the doctors needed to take it out, and 'mummy's hair maybe a bit funny after my operation'. All the while I was thinking, 'please God let it only be my hair.'

I went to Build a Bear and spent a small fortune - more than my wedding ring anyway - on two bears. They both had my voice in them saying mummy loved them. Yes, I did feel like a tit in the shop talking into a small microphone but my sons would love them I'm sure.

I researched cool places that we could spend a night away with The Stinks for a treat. I booked a night away in a converted helicopter. The Stinks would love that. Arguable, not the greatest idea when Adam is six feet five inches. It was cramped to say the least, and the next day Adam moaned about having a bad back. I thought, really Adam are you really trying to take the limelight off me? I think I trump your bad back with a brain tumour mate. I gave Ted and Albie their teddies, Ted was delighted, Albie hated it. He said he didn't like his voice. Cheers Albie. Each night when I put Albie to bed, I'd sneak the teddy with my voice in with him, but when

I went to check on him later in the night, the teddy was thrown on the floor with a barrage of nerf bullets all around him.

The night before the operation my mum and dad came for tea, which sadly had to be a non-greasy tea due to surgery the next day. I was being brave on the outside, then went into the kitchen and cried like a baby to my mum. No matter how old you are you always need your mum in a crisis and my mum was always there for me. My mum explained to me that if anything were to go wrong she would make sure Ted and Albie were always happy, and I wasn't to worry about them and just focus on getting better. In my head I was hoping for a quick stay in hospital then back to normal. That night I could have easily backed out.

The next morning Adam and I set off. I had planned my outfit, no surprise there. We arrived at the hospital at 6.30am. I was feeling okay, I was positive. Next, I was escorted into a cubicle, where I was asked the same questions by lots of different people, they drew an arrow on my neck pointing to my ear. That made me laugh, something as important as this and they were using a biro. I knew I was going to be deaf permanently in my left side after the operation, but I was seeing that as a positive in our crazy house.

Adam and I were making small talk trying to stay positive. 'Think about that dream home you've always wanted', Adam said, 'we will get that after you are better'. The anesthetist came in just in the middle of this conversation. Damn it, I needed to get Adam to give me a budget and a time frame, I needed these in writing before I went in. I was never going to get him to say these words again. Could I up my limit on my Right Move Search? All these unanswered questions.

I was escorted down to the theatre by a man wearing a bandana and a tattoo on his forearm with the words 'Wendy' on it. You forget nurses are real people and have a life outside of the theatre.

My operation was to take eight hours and bandana man would want to get home to Wendy just as much as I wanted to be home with The Stinks. When I walked down there I did think, bloody hell, the biggest surgery of my life and I have to walk to the theatre, but considering nothing was wrong with my legs, maybe it didn't justify a wheelchair. It did feel odd. I could have just turned and done a runner and Wendy's guy wouldn't have stood a chance.

I lay on the bed and a slow procession of tears rolled down my cheeks. I was shit scared. They waved what looked like an oxygen mask in my face and said I would feel sleepy. Shit it's not working, 'it's not working', I called out to the anesthetist. That was the last thing I remember.

Three things I am grateful for;

- **Feeling positive**
- **The great nurses, surgeons and staff at Salford Hope Hospital**
- **Getting Adam to 'sort of' commit to buying a bigger house**

Waking up Brianless

I was in the operating theatre for nine and a half hours, Albie was at playschool and didn't give me a second thought and Ted was at school then a cinema night straight afterwards in the school hall, his only concern was which film he was going to watch. And quite rightly too.

I woke up hearing Wendy's bloke saying, 'wake up Irene, smile for us.' Smile? Are you effing serious, I've just had brain surgery? I hazily explained to them I had been shopping in the Trafford Centre, a perfect dream for me. I grimaced a smile as much as I could, then they wheeled me out of theatre. My mum, dad and Adam were at my side, my lips were curled up in front of my teeth like Mr Ed the talking horse. Water, I needed water.

Worried about the facial nerve, I asked them 'how do I look? is my face okay?' to which my mum just said 'Irene, you look beautiful'. I fell asleep.

The next morning, I woke to numerous visitors, all of whom knew me, as they had seen inside my head, not metaphorically, but actually seen inside my head. But I didn't know them. 'Hi, I'm suchabody and I was in theatre with you.' This continued all day; I was very popular. I was so tempted to ask if anyone had taken a photo of my brain or a selfie of my brain and them while they were in there. I would have loved a photo, but Adam said I wasn't to ask for one. The surgeon arrived and explained they had removed all my tumour and hadn't touched the facial nerve.

My last visitor was an anesthetist I knew, one of the Dad's at Albie's preschool. He chatted for about five minutes then said, 'have you seen a mirror?' Panicked, I thought no why? what was I going to see. I was instantly worried. My heart started to pound but he went on, 'I'll take a photo and show you.' He showed me the photo. I had a massive bandage around my head and due to the way I'd been sleeping, it was half on, half off, tufts of hair sticking out. I looked like I had a Christmas party hat on half cut. How come not one of my visitors had told me? I felt like I had spent all day with a bogie on the end of my nose and no one had the balls to tell me. In the grand scheme of things, I got over it.

In my hospital bag I had taken a book about positivity, my make-up, a face mask and three lovely pairs of new Marks and Spencer's pyjamas. You can't go wrong with M&S PJs. I spent the four days I was in hospital in the same pair of PJs, slept all the time and never even brushed my teeth. Another expectation versus reality moment.

On the Thursday, the physiotherapist came to my bed to see if I could walk. If I could walk and climb the stairs I could go home. I know I would have felt better at home but the thought of having no nurses checking on me every thirty minutes just two days after major brain surgery seemed a little daunting. I walked very slowly, short steps whilst the physio held my arm. We arrived at the stairs and she asked me if my house had a bannister on the stairs. I couldn't remember - it was a bit like when you have been talking to someone for a while and when you try and describe them you can't remember if they had a moustache or glasses. I told her, 'no'.

Our town house, which was only eight years old, with two flights of stairs didn't have a bannister? Of course it had bannisters, but for the life of me I couldn't remember them. Because I'd said no, I wasn't allowed to hold the hand rail while I was attempting the stairs in the hospital that day. I failed to manage to walk down without help, so back to bed I went.

I was in a room with four other ladies and we all had a big dressing on some part of our head. I was the youngest by a fair few years and they all wanted to chat. All I wanted to do was sleep. I had to make the most of having no Stinks with me.

On the Friday I was allowed home. I had my going home outfit ready but decided to just stick a hoody over the top of my four days worn in PJs, spray some deodorant around me and pop some Wrigley's extra in. I slowly walked out of the hospital like a wounded animal, leaning on Adam for support in every way.

Once at the car I felt faint and overheated. Quickly, I wound down the window and put my hand out to get some breeze. Adam put his ticket in the car park machine and put both windows up, trapping my hand in the process. 'Agh!' I screamed. Adam panicked. He thought my head had come undone. 'My hand! My hand!'

'Ooops,' he said. I called him a muppet - or words to that effect.

Once home, with a throbbing head and now a throbbing hand too, I had the long process of getting better. Ted and Albie had been warned they couldn't jump on mummy; couldn't wake me up; couldn't shoot me with a Nerf gun. Ted took it all in his stride, however Albie had decided the best course of action was not to come near me at all. The temptation of a sly bullet in the head must have been too much …

Adam helped loads around the house and I realised that I was in a very good bargaining position.

Things I am grateful for;

- **Wendy's bloke**
- **Having a new collection of unworn pajamas**
- **Having a break from Nerf wars**

Back to Life, Back to Reality

I had always wanted a dog and both Ted and Albie loved animals. I had practised at being a pet owner in the past to show Adam I was competent, but I didn't quite cut it.

I once saw a poster outside Albie's pre-school asking for someone to help over the Easter holidays to look after Mr Stickman, it goes without saying he was a stick insect. I volunteered, Albie would be so pleased taking Mr Stickman home and he can write all about his stay with us over the holidays. All I had to do was clear out his bed, and feed him leaves, he died two days before he was due back. Adam searched the internet looking to get a replacement before the spring term started. I have a photo of Albie proudly taking back Mr Stickman II - oblivious. I didn't volunteer again. Strangely, they didn't ask me again either.

Adam was still reluctant for us to have a dog. I decided to get a cat, they were easy to look after, weren't they? I'm not a cat lover, but I wouldn't harm one. Our kitten arrived and was named Tickles. Albie loved Tickles. The feeling wasn't mutual. After around six months, Tickles got run over. Personally, I think he may have taken his own life after living in our house.   I had to tell the lads. I googled how to tell a young person a pet has died. Straight to the point. Okay, I sat them down. I explained Tickles had been run over and was now in heaven. Ted started to cry which made me cry. Albie said, 'so is he flat?'

'Yes Albie, he is flat.'

Ted cried louder, then after a few minutes, Ted asked what car was it that ran him over. Unsure as to what to say, I said it

115

was a small car. Phew it the right answer. Ted seemed to find solace in the fact that it was a small car. Albie asked for a new cat now Tickles was flat.

A short time later we did get another cat and let Albie name it. The cat is called Flip Flop.

As I was now in recovery now would be the perfect time to get a dog. I begged and pleaded and eventually Barney arrived. Albie didn't get a choice on names this time. Barney is a small Cavachon. Which to me means he is a mongrel, apparently the correct term now is that he's a cross bread.

I read all I could about having a dog I didn't want to fail again. I had a dog den built under the stairs by my handy man - not Adam - and bought Barney plenty of coats and a bow tie. What else did he need?

Barney settled in very well, I've had a few 5am get ups, which Adam refuses to do. He said I wanted the dog, so I can deal with him. I wanted the children so does that mean I have to deal with them too?

We've recently introduced Ted to cricket, we did football previously, but it didn't work out. We try to take them to watch cricket as Adam loves it and I like the atmosphere. When we first started going, I liked the idea of sitting in the sun drinking wine and not being judged. I drink pop now. We took Barney the dog to his first cricket match. Other people have their dogs there, what's the worst that can happen? Adam went to the bar while Ted, Albie, Barney and I found a bench near the front of the spectators' area. As I was still in recovery and didn't leave the house much, I decided to wash my face and make an effort. Lovely summer dress on and wedges. Barney wanted to play. He wriggled that much that he escaped his harness and ran onto the pitch. 'Quick, Ted, get him.' Ted just looked at me gormlessly. Great. I ran down the grass embankment, went over on my ankle broke my expensive eBay wedges. The ankle strap still attached, I dropped to the floor like a sack of shit. Eventually I got the ankles straps off and ran across the pitch in my bare feet. Adam walked back from the bar to see me walking across the pitch with Barney in my arms, no shoes and a sweaty head. He just shook his head. I love these relaxing family times.

We have tried to get Ted interested in many different activities and spent a small fortune in the process. He started at a football club at eighteen months, but I stopped going, getting there for 9am on a Sunday morning just to have Ted run in the opposite direction to all the other children didn't seem that appealing, never mind paying for the privilege too.

He tried guitar lessons. Adam loved to play the guitar and would love for Ted and Albie to follow in his footsteps. I played the clarinet as a child. Father Christmas brought me one, I started lessons, but quickly realised it was my not forte. I had other interests instead, like boys and clothes. I sold my clarinet for £15 so I could buy myself a pair of shell suit trousers; I couldn't afford the top.

Ted's guitar teacher clearly hadn't taught anyone as young as Ted, he would strum some notes, then look at Ted. Ted in turn would look blankly at me. I noted the teacher hadn't asked Ted to copy him, so it was down to me to say to Ted, now you play it. The lessons went on pretty much in the same vein each week. In a half hour lesson not much was achieved. Ted said he wanted to stop his lessons and he tried again when he was ten. A bit precise but okay.

We went to Karate. At first, we thought we had found the one. Full kit and insurance purchased to then realise we had maybe peaked too early as most of Ted's Karate techniques he looked more like a contemporary dancer on acid.

Ted then started Beavers. Adam was in the Scouts and has fond memories. He talks about being in the scouts in some way veterans talk about their deployments. I've been told on many occasions how he was kicked out of scouts like he was some sort of rebel without a cause. On Ted's first session, he skipped out beaming - they had been sewing all evening. I think we have found Ted's calling.

His first badge was for a swimming gala, I was slightly apprehensive as he wasn't a brilliant swimmer even though we had paid for lessons since he was ten weeks old.

What Ted lacks in ability he certainly makes up for in enthusiasm. He volunteered to swim the back-stroke heat. He has never even done back stroke. Adam and I sat in the spectator seats high up. I wanted to be cool but as soon as the starter pistol was fired, I started shouting like a banshee. Ted was on his back, arms flaying all over. Ted beaming, looking up at us. All the other parents stopped shouting as their child had finished but Ted was still only half way. I continued to shout out his name, I couldn't let him do another half to no-one shouting and cheering. Ted looked to his left and to his right and didn't see anyone. His smiled widened, he thought he was winning. My heart broke for him. I think the other parents felt sorry for him as they all started calling his name and cheering him on. Ted got out of the pool and gave me a big thumbs up and then the realisation came over him that all the other swimmers were sat down waiting for him to finish, and his thumb turned down. He was devastated.

Give him his due he continued to volunteer for every race he could. He didn't get any medals, but he got his first badge and that's all that mattered.

He recently went on a Beavers' camp for one night. As I was driving him there, I thought I should be passing on some words of wisdom for him. I wracked my brain trying to think of anything useful. In the end I blurted out 'Remember, Ted, what's in your underpants is private'. Great mothering skills, Irene.

We've decided to take a different path with Albie and just let him tell us what he wants to do. The only hobby coming through so far is Nerf Gun shooting. Hmmm?

Three things I am grateful for;

- **All stink insects look the same**
- **Getting our new addition Barney to add to our crazy family**
- **Ted showing us that he has determination**

Finally getting my 'Carrie Bradshaw' back

My recovery was basically sleep. They say your brain goes into shock after surgery. Mine did, think of baby brain and times that by ten. I was told to sleep and rest most of the time and listen to my body. I was so impressed with myself when I went out for lunch with Adam ten days after brain surgery but that one hour in a restaurant lead to three-hour nap when I got home.

Everybody I saw said I looked amazing …considering, I didn't read too much into the last part.

I had an appointment to go to see the community nurse two weeks after my operation to have the staples in my stomach removed where they had removed the fat. Don't get me wrong, I won't be in a bikini anytime soon, and I already have a scar from two c-sections, but for some reason I had expected they would be do key hole surgery to suck the fact out. I was a bit shocked to find fifteen stables going across my stomach and now my curved stomach had a corner on the left side.

The nurse had what appeared to be plyers in her hand to cut the staples and already I was tensed up, but I didn't feel a thing. Brain surgery must have made me hard as nails. I didn't even realise she'd started when she said all done.

My scar on my head goes all around my ear then slightly down my neck. I'm proud of this scar. It's like wearing a t shirt when you have run a marathon, telling the world, 'look what I survived'. Although for my brain surgery, all I had to do was go to sleep for ten hours, not actually do any running, thank God.

Hannah came home for a week and we spent a week together. Now Hannah is older, we have so much in common. I wish I had been as clued up on things when I was her age. Me, Catherine and Hannah all went out together and we realised that was the first time the three of us had actually gone out together.

Hannah is more like me than Catherine. She loves planning, lists, a good journal, positivity but she is a romantic. She reads and has read classic novels since she was ditched on our nights out. She had a choice whether to go to Paris the city or Disneyland Paris when she was seven and she chose the city. Even though there are twenty years between Hannah and I, she just slotted into the sisterhood perfectly. I feel a bit sorry for my dad because when we are all together with my mum, he doesn't get a look in. I don't think he understands us, as we start a sentence and without finishing it, all fall about laughing. It's quite hard to get into our clique. But I love our clique.

I had been given a list of do's and don'ts by the hospital - if brain fluid started leaking from my nose or my wound, then I was to go straight back in. Don't worry, I wouldn't have been waiting around …

Thankfully, nothing liked that happened. I lost my taste buds on my tongue, but as I am basically used to inhaling my food, I didn't really use them anyway. The, being deaf on one side has taken a bit of getting used to. To over-compensate for not hearing things, if Adam and I were watching TV, I'd turn to him and say, 'sorry, what did you say?'

He'd reply, 'I didn't say anything'. After I had asked him about ten times, he lost his rag so now I don't say it anymore.

If it's important, I'm sure he'll make sure I hear him. I suspect he is possibly using this to his advantage though, as now when he tells me when he's setting off on a night out to watch a band, he'll say, 'OMG, I've told you all about this about ten times'. Hmm, I'm not too sure.

It's funny when we are in the 'throes of passion' and he'll lean into my left ear and I'll have to say, 'if you've just said something, you're going to have to use my other ear'. Sort of takes the sexiness out of it.

In my list of do's and don'ts was don't strain, which included sneezing. How do you stop yourself from sneezing? I had visions of sneezing and my brain popping out. Also, the straining included having a number two. Maybe a bit too much detail, but I've told you everything else about me. If you've ever had anaesthetic you are pretty blocked up for the first couple of days and the first time you go, it's like giving birth. Well, imagine that and trying not to strain your head. I had to hold onto the left side of my head in a bid to keep my brain inside.

I slowly got back into exercising. Pre-kids and pre-Brian I was a bit of a gym-bunny, I would do two classes a night after eating just a banana all day, then stop for some wine and ten fags on the way home. I was the skinniest I'd ever been, granted probably not the healthiest.

I've had a gym membership every year since I was eighteen. After Albie was born and I realised I had post-natal depression, I started the couch to 5K. It was just what I needed at the time, for my mental health as much as my physical health. However, I hate running. I had the same play list every time and eventually managed to run 5k - twice. Then I stopped.

I've heard that athletes use a method in training where they visualise competing and how they feel at certain parts in their race and it has the same effect as doing the race itself, so I keep playing the playlist that I used for the couch to 5K, and visualise running up our road, but my arse is still fat. How does it work for athletes and not me? I've decided to do things now that I actually enjoy, like Zumba and street dance. Another dream of mine was to be a backing dancer on Top of the Pops. Hmm, I might pop that on my goal board.

I re-did my goal board. Adam usually sniggers at me when I'm doing this but it wasn't long before he stuck a couple of goals on there for himself. Not a stupid idea now is it, Adam? Although when I sat back to admire my handy work, I sat on the glass front of my goal-board that I had placed on the sofa. 'Jesus Christ', I jumped up, 'What the hell was that?' and saw all the pieces of glass. As I am now in my positive place, I've taken it as a sign that I am going to smash my goals, just glad I didn't end up with splinters in my arse.

I started meditating and trying to do things which improved our wellbeing as a family. I was on a mission. I was fully focused on living my life. I tried to involve Adam and kids as much as possible. We headed out one evening walking the dog and I told them all we were going to be silent for sixty seconds and let's just listen and appreciate the sounds we can hear. Thirty seconds in and it all became too much. Albie was the first to squeeze a pump out, then Ted, followed by Adam. They all rolled around in fits of laughter. When Ted and Albie were struggling to force more out, I thought, this is going to take a serious turn for the worse, so we decided to just go back to chatting. I tried.

Whilst off recuperating we were invited to my step brother's wedding. We took The Stinks with us as it was nice to go out as a family. Albie and Ted ran around the venue like crazed animals. They pillaged the sweet cart and left scraps for the other children. In his E-number induced haze, Albie went to the toilet. He'd been gone a while (he's now at the age he refuses to come into the ladies with me). Adam went to investigate. Ted then went to investigate as both Adam and Albie hadn't returned. Ted came running back to me and said, a man was stood on the radiator in the toilets. Oh no! I had no idea what was going on, but I sure as hell knew that it involved Albie. Yep, sure enough Albie was locked in the cubicle and there were about five men trying to get him out. Eventually - after the groom had his best man balanced on his shoulder trying to climb over - they had to get the staff in and break the door down.

Albie walked out, as cool as a cucumber and fist-bumped all the men who had come to his rescue. Home time I think.

That's why we don't venture out as a family often.

I spent a few of weeks watching back-to-back Say Yes to the Dress. After about a month, I was going insane. I was still very tired but when I did have energy spurts I got my lap top out and continued to write again.

When life-changing things happen to you, it makes you look at things differently. I never wanted to live to work or just plod along complaining that things are always the same. I have learnt that there are certain things you have no control over but the things you do have control over, grab by the balls and do something about them. I enjoy my job, don't get me wrong, and I know Adam enjoys his but we both had things we always wanted to do. Adam, being into his music, always wanted to DJ. I decided to buy him a mixing desk, before he lost all his hair and look like an aging rocker, and I got serious with my book. I always wanted to write. I always wanted to be a public speaker too and hopefully help people in the process. Every bit of energy I had, when the kids were at school, was now spent on bettering myself. I listened to lots more self-help books, how to public speak books, how to be an author books, along with my 'quit lit'. Now I wasn't drinking wine I had a few spare hours to fill and extra brain cells to use.

When you count up the hours you have in a week, there are one hundred and sixty-eight. Say you work forty of those hours, that leaves one hundred and twenty eight, then add in sleep (and I need a good eight hours a night), that leaves fifty-six hours. Fifty-six hours is a lot of time: time to spend with your family, follow your dreams, make plans, learn new things or just sleep some more, but I planned to make the most of them.

Every half an hour or so I'd remember something I'd like to add into my book. My iPhone notes was full of random words to jog my memory when I got the laptop out. Before I knew it, I'd written ten thousand words. That was just emptying my head and I loved it. I needed to know if I was barking up the wrong tree. Was I delusional and should I stick to buying bankruptcy stock?? I got in touch with a writer and sent out an extract from what I had written. The anxiety/excitement was massive, if this was shite there was only me responsible. With the Aloe Vera phase if someone didn't like the product it wasn't a personal dig, but now I am bearing all and waiting for feedback. I was the product...

When I got the feedback I was spurred on. I felt positive about life and it gave me confidence in what I was doing. Don't get me wrong, I realise I'm no J K Rowling, but I was happy with where I was. Writing really seemed to balance me; any thoughts, rational or irrational, I unloaded onto paper or my laptop and they seemed to be a lot clearer once out of my head.

As I went on, I realised that this could be the positive from Dusty. I would only have dreamed about writing a book before I had Dusty but having him had changed me. I talk about Ted and Albie all the time and I wanted to talk about Dusty as much as I do my other sons. This is the way I could do this.

I decided to go one step further and tell anyone who would listen about Dusty and our life. I started putting myself out there as a public speaker. This was way out of my comfort zone, but suddenly I came alive, I felt butterflies in my stomach, I couldn't decide if it was anxiety or excitement about where our lives were going. But whatever it was I liked the feeling. Plus, on the positive side to that, my Fitbit said I was most days in fat-burning mode just with this feeling inside me. Bonus.

After my first public speaking event, which I thoroughly enjoyed after the first ten minutes of dry mouth and shaky hands subsided, I realised that I had been given these things in my life because I am strong. I have stopped thinking, that because I have been strong once, I don't need to be tested again. I refuse to be a victim of life. I may be tested again, but I know now that I can handle anything life throws at me and in time, I will be okay again.

My next MRI scan is February 2021 and if the sucker decides he wants to come back then I am ready for him.

I read about the five second rule by Mel Robbins, and basically thought, fuck it and just do it, to anything that scared me or that I would normally have put off. At the same time this pushed me a little bit closer to my dreams. It wasn't always big steps - little steps forward make a happy life.

There were times I would doubt myself and still do. I researched Imposter Syndrome. Who was I kidding? Who did I think I was? Was I going to make the difference that I wanted to make? But if just one person listens to me, or reads this, and I have helped them get through tough times, then that's my difference made. If it is more than one person, that's even better.

When I was researching for this book I looked at some statistics. The chances of having a still born baby are scarily 1 in 200, the chances of having the type of brain tumour I had is 1 in 200,000, the chances of having both these plus drinking your child's pee is about one in a million - that part wasn't on Google strangely enough.

I'm not saying I'm special, but I am unique, as we all are. We all have our own story, whether we decide to say it out loud, write it down or keep it to ourselves. I hope you've enjoyed my story.

'Look up to the sky.
You'll never find the rainbows if you're looking down'

Things I am grateful for;

My LIFE

Lightning Source UK Ltd.
Milton Keynes UK
UKHW021110300821
389711UK00013B/1118